DEMONSTRATING YOUR COMPETENCE 3: CARDIOVASCULAR AND NEUROLOGICAL CONDITIONS

Gill Wakley
Ruth Chambers
and
Simon Ellis

RADCLIFFE MEDICAL PRESS
Oxford • San Francisco

Radcliffe Publishing Ltd
18 Marcham Road
Abingdon
Oxon OX14 1AA
United Kingdom

www.radcliffe-oxford.com
Electronic catalogue and worldwide online ordering.

British Library Cataloguing in Publication Data

A catalogue record for this book is available from the British Library.

ISBN 1 85775 843 9

Typeset by Advance Typesetting Ltd, Oxfordshire
Printed and bound by T J International Ltd, Padstow, Cornwall

Contents

Preface

The General Medical Council has asked doctors to start thinking now about how they will collect and keep the information that will show that they should continue to hold a licence to practise as doctors from 2005 onwards. The onus will be on individual doctors to show that they are up to date and fit to practise medicine throughout their careers. It will be doctors who decide for themselves the nature of the information they collect and retain that best reflects their roles and responsibilities in their everyday work.

This book is the third of a series that will guide you as a general practitioner (GP) through the process, giving you examples and ideas as to how to document your learning, competence, performance or standards of service delivery. Chapter 1 explains the link between your personal development plans, local appraisal and the revalidation of your medical registration. Learning and service improvements that are integral to your personal development plan are central to the documents that you include in your appraisal and revalidation portfolio.

The stages of the evidence cycle that we suggest are built upon the underpinning publication: Chambers R, Wakley G, Field S and Ellis S (2003) *Appraisal for the Apprehensive*. Radcliffe Medical Press, Oxford.

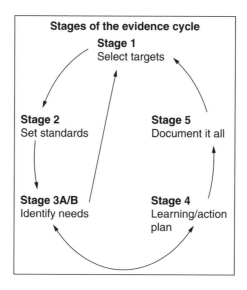

Stage 1 is about setting targets or aspirations for good practice. Many of the aspirations we suggest are taken from *Good Medical Practice*[1] or its sister publication, *Good Medical Practice for General Practitioners*.[2] Stage 2 encourages you as a professional to set standards for the outcomes of what you plan to learn more about, or outcomes relating to you providing a good service in your practice.

Chapter 2 describes a variety of methods to help you to address Stage 3 of the cycle of evidence, to find out what it is you need to learn about or what gaps there are in the way you deliver care as an individual GP or as a team. This chapter includes a wide variety of methods doctors might use in their everyday work to identify and document these needs. One of the drivers for the introduction of appraisal and revalidation has been to reassure the public and others of doctors' continuing fitness to practise. So it makes sense that we have emphasised the importance of obtaining feedback from patients in this chapter in relation to identifying your learning and service development needs.

Best practice in addressing the giving of informed consent by patients, maintaining confidentiality of patient information and organising responsive complaints processes are all common components of good quality healthcare. Chapter 3 covers these aspects in depth and provides the first example of cycles of evidence for you to consider adopting or adapting for your own circumstances. The focus of each cycle of evidence is on one of the 'headings' from *Good Medical Practice*[1] or the standard appraisal format.

The rest of the book consists of seven clinically based chapters that span key topics in cardiovascular and neurological conditions. The first part of each chapter covers key issues that are likely to crop up in typical consultations for each clinical field. The second part of each chapter gives examples of cycles of evidence in a similar format to those in Chapter 3.

Overall, you will probably want to choose three or four cycles of evidence each year. You might choose one or two from Chapter 3 and the rest from clinical areas such as those covered by Chapters 4 to 10. You might like this way of learning and service development so much that you build up a bigger bank of evidence, taking one cycle from each chapter in the same year. Whatever your approach, you will want to keep your cycles of evidence as short and simple as possible, so that the documentation itself is a by-product of the learning and action plans you undertake to improve the service you provide, and does not dominate your time and effort at work.

While you are establishing your professional competence, you will also be recording the information to substantiate your practice claims for quality payments. Information will be extracted using Read codes from software designed to search for the relevant domains. Quality markers can only be confirmed by the data recorded on the computer system. Registers of patients with the relevant conditions must be accurate, so invest time in confirming that those people recorded as, for example, suffering from heart failure actually have it. Many of the indicators of quality overlap – for example, recording blood pressure, smoking, smoking cessation and influenza immunisation – and can be counted in more than one clinical area. The maximum points will be staged according to the percentage of patients gradually included in the target figures. The percentages given in the relevant chapters are the maximum to aim for, not those that will be achieved in the first year!

Other books in the series are based on the same format of the five stages in the cycle of evidence. Book 1 helps doctors and other health professionals to demonstrate that they are competent teachers or trainers, and the following books set out key information and examples of evidence for a wide variety of clinical areas for GPs and other doctors.

This approach and style of learning will take a bit of getting used to for doctors. Until now, they have not had to prove that they are fit to practise unless the General Medical Council has investigated them for a significant reason such as a complaint or error. Until recently, most doctors did not evaluate what they learnt or whether they applied it in practice. They did not protect time for learning and reflection among their everyday responsibilities, or target their time and effort on priority topics. Times are changing, and with the introduction of personal development plans and appraisal GPs are realising that they must take a more professional approach to learning, and document their standards of competence, performance and service delivery. This book helps them to do just that.

Please note that resources to support this book are provided at http://health.mattersonline.net.

References

1   General Medical Council (2001) *Good Medical Practice*. General Medical Council, London.

2   Royal College of General Practitioners/General Practitioners' Committee (2002) *Good Medical Practice for General Practitioners*. Royal College of General Practitioners, London.

About the authors

Gill Wakley started in general practice but transferred to community medicine shortly afterwards and then into public health. A desire for increased contact with patients caused a move back into general practice. She has been heavily involved in learning and teaching throughout her career. She was in a training general practice, became an instructing doctor and a regional assessor in family planning, and was until recently a senior clinical lecturer with the Primary Care Department at Keele University. Like Ruth, she has run all types of educational initiatives and activities. A visiting professor at Staffordshire University, she now works as a freelance GP, writer and lecturer.

Ruth Chambers has been a GP for more than 20 years and is currently the head of the Stoke-on-Trent Teaching Primary Care Trust programme and professor of primary care development at Staffordshire University. Ruth has worked with the Royal College of General Practitioners to enable GPs to gather evidence about their learning and standards of practice while striving to be excellent GPs. Ruth has co-authored a series of books with Gill, designed to help readers draw up their own personal development plans or workplace learning plans around key clinical topics.

Simon Ellis has been a constant neurologist at the University Hospital of North Staffordshire for ten years where he runs the neurovascular (TIA) clinic. He is a visiting professor in neurosciences at Staffordshire University. He has been involved in medical education, both undergraduate and graduate, for many years and runs a session on appraisal for medical educators. He has published on general neurology, appraisal and epilepsy.

1

Making the link: personal development plans, appraisal and revalidation

The nexus of personal development plans, appraisal and revalidation

Learning involves many steps. It includes the acquisition of information, its retention, the ability to retrieve the information when needed and how to use that information for best practice. Demonstrating your learning involves being able to show the steps you have taken. Learning should be lifelong and encompass continuing professional development.

Continuing professional development (CPD) takes time. It makes sense to utilise the time spent by overlapping learning to meet your personal and professional needs, with that required for the performance of your role in the health service.

Many doctors have drawn up a personal development plan (PDP) that is agreed with their local CPD or college tutor. Some doctors have constructed their PDP in a systematic way and identified the priorities within it, or gathered evidence to demonstrate that what they learnt about was subsequently applied in practice. Tutors do not have a uniform approach to the style and relevance of a doctor's PDP. Some are content that a plan has been drawn up, while others encourage the doctor to develop a systematic approach to identifying and addressing their learning and service needs, in order of importance or urgency.[1]

The new emphasis on doctors' accountability to the public has given the PDP a higher profile and shown that it may be used in other ways. The medical education establishment and NHS management argue about the balance between its alternative uses. The educationalists view a PDP as a tool to encourage doctors to plan their own learning activities. The management view is of a tool allowing quality assurance of the doctor's performance. Doctors, striving to improve the quality of the care that they deliver to patients, want to use a PDP to guide them on their way, perhaps towards postgraduate awards of universities or the quality awards of the Royal College of General

Practitioners (RCGP). These quality awards are built around the standards of excellence to which a general practitioner (GP) should aspire, as described in the publication, *Good Medical Practice for General Practitioners*.[2]

Your personal development plan

Your PDP will be an integral part of your future appraisal and revalidation portfolio to demonstrate your fitness to practise as a doctor.

Your initial plan should:

*   identify your gaps or weaknesses in knowledge, skills or attitudes
*   specify topics for learning as a result of changes: in your role, responsibilities, the organisation in which you work
*   link into the learning needs of others in your workplace or team of colleagues
*   tie in with the service development priorities of your practice, the primary care organisation (PCO) or the NHS as a whole
*   describe how you identified your learning needs
*   set your learning needs and associated goals in order of importance and urgency
*   justify your selection of learning goals
*   describe how you will achieve your goals and over what time period
*   describe how you will evaluate learning outcomes.

Each year you will continue or revise your PDP. It should demonstrate how you carried out your learning and evaluation plans, show that you have learnt what you set out to do (or why it was modified) and how you applied your new learning in practice. In addition, you will find that you have new priorities and fresh learning needs as circumstances change.

The main task is to capture what you have learnt, in a way that suits you. Then you can look back at what you have done and:

*   reflect on it later, to decide to learn more, or to make changes as a result, and identify further needs
*   demonstrate to others that you are fit to practise or work through:
    *   what you have done
    *   what you have learnt
    *   what changes you have made as a result
    *   the standards of work you have achieved and are maintaining
    *   how you monitor your performance at work
*   use it to show how your personal learning fits in with the requirements of your practice or the NHS, and other people's personal and professional development plans.

Organise all the evidence of your learning into a continuing professional development portfolio of some sort. It is up to you how you keep this record of your learning. Examples are:

- *an ongoing learning journal* in which you draw up and describe your plan, record how you determined your needs and prioritised them, report why you attended particular educational meetings or courses and what you got out of them as well as the continuing cycle of review, making changes and evaluating them
- *an A4 file* with lots of plastic sleeves into which you build up a systematic record of your educational activities in line with your plan
- *a box*: chuck in everything to do with your learning plan as you do it and sort it out into a sensible order every few months with a good review once a year.

The context of appraisal and revalidation

Appraisal and revalidation are based on the same sources of information – presented in the same structure as the headings set out in the General Medical Council (GMC) guidance in *Good Medical Practice*.[3] The two processes perform different functions. Whereas revalidation involves an assessment against a standard of fitness to practise medicine, appraisal is concerned with the doctor's professional development within his or her working environment and the needs of the organisation for which the doctor works.

Appraisal is a formative and developmental process that is being introduced by the Departments of Health for all GPs and hospital consultants working in the NHS across the UK. While the details of the appraisal system vary for consultants and GPs and for each of the countries, the educational principles remain the same. The aims of the appraisal system are to give doctors an opportunity to discuss and receive regular feedback on their previous and continuing performance and identify education and development needs.

The drive to introduce formal appraisals came initially as part of the programme to introduce clinical governance across the NHS as laid out in the 1998 consultation document *A First Class Service*.[4] Momentum was gained with the publication of *Supporting Doctors, Protecting Patients* (1999) in England which outlined a set of proposals to help prevent doctors from developing problems.[5] Appraisal was at the heart of the proposals as:

a positive process to give someone feedback on their performance, to chart their continuing progress and to identify development needs. It is a forward looking process essential for the developmental and educational planning needs of an individual. *Assessment* is the process of measuring progress against agreed criteria ... It is not the primary aim of appraisal to scrutinise doctors to see if they are performing poorly but rather to help them consolidate and improve on good performance aiming towards excellence.[5]

The document went on to suggest that appraisal should be made comprehensive and compulsory for doctors working in the NHS and form part of a future revalidation system.

In addition, appraisal should also address other areas of particular importance to the individual doctor. A standardised approach has been developed which utilises approved documentation. This should ensure that information from a variety of NHS employers is recorded consistently. The format of the paperwork is slightly different for consultants and GPs.

Appraisal must be a positive, formative and developmental process to support high quality patient care and improve clinical standards. Appraisal is different from, but linked to, revalidation.[6] Revalidation is the process whereby doctors will be regularly required to demonstrate that they are fit to practise. Appraisal feeds into this by contributing to the information that a doctor supplies for the revalidation process. Appraisal will provide a regular structured recording system for documenting progress towards revalidation and identifying needs as part of the doctor's PDP. Both the NHS appraisal and the revalidation structures are based on the same seven headings set out in the GMC's guidance *Good Medical Practice.*[3] The GMC claims, therefore, that 'five satisfactory appraisals equals revalidation'.[6] The GMC has also pledged that doctors not taking part in appraisal will be able to provide their own information for revalidation, providing this evidence meets the same criteria as in *Good Medical Practice.*[3]

Appraisal is, however, a two-way process. Not only time, but also resources will be needed to make appraisal systems successful. In addition, appraisal will identify issues that will require extra investment by the NHS in the educational and organisational infrastructure.

Appraisal and revalidation processes are being increasingly integrated. The PDP is a central part of the appraisal documentation, which will in turn be included in the portfolio of information available for revalidation. It seems that the evolution will continue so that revalidation is met by supporting the appraisal documentation with additional documents about clinical governance activity and CPD. These supporting documents will be a mix of subjective and objective information that will include doctors' self-assessment of their performance and other work-based assessment.

The revalidation and appraisal processes need to be quality assured to be able to demonstrate that they can protect the public from poor or underperforming doctors. Such quality assurance will relate to the appraisers, their training and support, as well as systems to examine the quality of evidence in the documentation relating to a doctor's performance and outcomes of their PDP. You should regard your PDP and supporting documentation as central to the way in which you can show, to anyone who requires you to do so, that your performance as a doctor is acceptable and that you are trying to improve, or striving for excellence.

Demonstrating the standards of your practice

The GMC sets out standards that must be met as part of the duties and responsibilities of doctors in the booklet *Good Medical Practice*.[3] Doctors must be able to meet these standards with a record of their own performance in their revalidation portfolio if they want to retain a licence to practise. The nine key headings of expected standards of practice for all GPs working in England are shown in Box 1.1.

Box 1.1:   Key headings of expected standards of practice for GPs working in England

1   *Good professional practice*. This relates to clinical care, keeping records (including writing reports and keeping colleagues informed), access and availability, treatment in emergencies and making effective use of resources.

2   *Maintaining good medical practice*. This includes keeping up to date and maintaining your performance.

3   *Relationships with patients*. This encompasses providing information about your services, maintaining trust, avoiding discrimination and prejudice against patients, relating well to patients and apologising if things go wrong.

4   *Working with colleagues.* This relates to working with colleagues, working in teams, referring patients and accepting posts.

5   *Teaching and training, appraising and assessing.* You may be in a position to teach or train colleagues or students, and appraise or assess peers, employees or students.

6   *Probity* includes providing true information about your services, honesty in financial and commercial dealings, and providing references.

7   *Health* can include how you overcome or compensate for health problems in yourself, or help with or address health problems in other doctors.

8   *Research.* Conducting research in an ethical manner.

9   *Management.* The section on management concerns any responsibility GPs have for management outside the practice. GPs might wish to include management responsibilities that cross the interface between their practice and PCO.

The appraisal paperwork for GPs working in England, Scotland, Wales and Northern Ireland has been individualised by each country. The English version for example, includes two extra sections to those of hospital consultants, management and research. The Scottish version focuses on core categories in preparation for revalidation of prescribing, referrals and peer review, clinical audit, significant event analysis and communication skills, summary of any complaints and other feedback.

The stages of the evidence cycle for demonstrating your standards of practice or competence and any necessary improvements are given in Figure 1.1. The stages of the evidence cycle are common to all the various areas of expertise considered in this book and will be followed in each chapter.

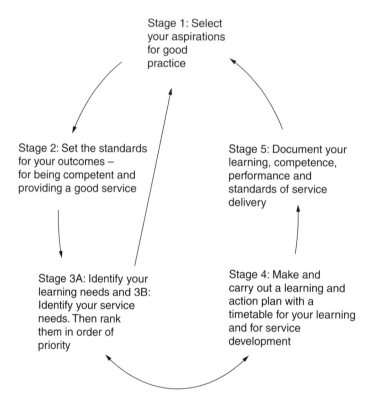

Figure 1.1:   Stages of the evidence cycle.

Although the five stages are shown in sequence here, in practice you would expect to move backwards and forwards from stage to stage, because of new information or a modification of your earlier ideas. New information might accrue when research is published which affects your clinical behaviour or standards, or a critical incident or patient complaint might occur which causes you and others to think anew about your standards or the way that services are delivered. The arrows in Figure 1.1 show that you might reset your target or aspirations for good practice, having undertaken exercises to identify what you need to learn or determine whether there are gaps in service delivery and, if so, what they are.

We suggest that you demonstrate your competence in focused areas of your day-to-day work by completing several cycles of evidence drawn from a variety of clinical or other areas each year, with at least one cycle of evidence from each of the main headings of *Good Medical Practice* over a five-year cycle.[3] By demonstrating your standards of practice around the main sections of *Good Medical Practice*, you will document your competence and performance for your revalidation portfolio in the same format as that required for your appraisal paperwork.

As you start to collate information about this five-stage cycle, discuss any problems about the standards of care or services you are looking at, with colleagues, experts in this area, tutors, etc. You want to develop a wide range and depth of evidence so that you can show that you are competent in your day-to-day general work as well as for any special areas of expertise.

Professional competence is the first area of concern in *Good Medical Practice*.[3] You should be able to demonstrate that you can maintain a satisfactory standard of clinical care most of the time in your everyday work. Some of the time you will be brilliant, of course! Celebrate those moments. On other occasions, you or others will be critical of your performance and feel that you could have done much better. Reflect on those episodes to learn from them.

Stage 1: Select your aspirations for good practice

By adopting or adapting descriptions of what an 'excellent' GP should be aiming for, you are defining the standards of practice for which all doctors should be aiming. The medical Royal Colleges have interpreted *Good Medical Practice* in various ways for the specialities of their own members.[3] For example, *Good Medical Practice for General Practitioners* describes the standards of practice that should be achieved by 'excellent' or 'unacceptable' GPs. Their definition of excellence is being 'consistently good'.[2]

This consistency is a critical factor in considering competence and performance too (*see* page 15). The documents that you collect in your evidence cycles must reflect consistency over time and in different circumstances, for example with various types of patients or your practice at different times of day. This will show that you have not only performed well on one occasion or for one type of baseline assessment, but also sustained your performance over time and under different conditions.

Stage 2: Set the standards for your outcomes – for being competent and providing a good service

Outcomes might include:

- the way that learning is applied
- a learnt skill
- a protocol
- a strategy that is implemented
- meeting recommended standards.

The level at which you should be performing depends on your particular field of expertise. GPs are good at seeing the wider picture, while specialists tend to be expert in a narrow area, so that the level of competence expected for a clinical area will vary depending on the doctor's role and responsibilities. You would not, for example, expect orthopaedic specialists to be competent at managing cardiac failure (although some of them may be), but you would expect GPs to be able to manage all but the most complicated situations involving cardiac failure. You would expect both the orthopaedic specialist and the GP to recognise the limits of their competence and to refer to someone with more expertise when necessary.

Other standards include using resources effectively and the record keeping that is an essential tool in clinical care. As a health professional, you need to be accessible and available so that you can provide your services, and make suitable arrangements for handing over care to others. You must provide care in an emergency.

You could incorporate into your standards or outcomes those components specified by universities at a national level as part of their Masters' Frameworks for their postgraduate awards. The Masters' Frameworks consist of eight components that shape the individual postgraduate award programme outcomes and the learning outcomes of the individual modules for the postgraduate awards. The eight components are shown in Box 1.2. You could set out your CPD work in the portfolio you are assembling for revalidation and your annual appraisals in this format. This would help you to document your professional development to date in a form that can be readily 'accredited for prior experiential learning' (APEL) by universities (contact your local universities if you want more information about this process). You might then be given credits for learning against an intended postgraduate award. It would save you from duplicating work as well as speeding your progress through the award.

If you have information or data about your practice showing that it was substandard or that you were not competent, you might choose to exclude that from your portfolio. However, you will be able to show that you have

---

Box 1.2:   The eight components of the Masters' Frameworks for postgraduate awards

1 Analysis
2 Problem solving
3 Knowledge and understanding
4 Reflection
5 Communication
6 Learning
7 Application
8 Enquiry

---

learnt more by reviewing mistakes or negative episodes. It is better to include everything of relevance, then go on to demonstrate how you addressed the gaps in your performance and made sustained improvements. You will need to protect the confidentiality of patients and colleagues as necessary when you collect data. The GMC will be seeing the contents of your revalidation portfolio if your submission is one of those sampled. You will probably also submit or share the documentation for appraisal and maybe use it for reviews with colleagues or the PCO.

Stage 3: Identify your learning and service needs in your practice or primary care organisation and rank them in order of priority[1]

The type and depth of documentation you need to gather will encompass:

• the context in which you work
• your knowledge and skills in relation to any particular role or responsibility of your current post.

The extent of expertise you should possess will depend on your level of responsibility for a particular function or task. You may be personally responsible for that function or task, or you may contribute or delegate responsibility for it. Your learning needs should take into account your aspirations for the future too – personal or career development for you, or improvements in the way you deliver care in your practice. Look at Chapter 2 for more ideas on how you will identify your learning or service development needs.

   Group and summarise your service development needs from the exercises you have carried out. Grade them according to the priority you set. You may put one at a higher priority because it fits in with service development needs established in the business plan of the trust or practice, or put another lower because it does not fit in with other activities that your organisation has in their current development plan for the next 12 months. If you have identified a service development need by several different methods of assessment or with several different patient groups or clinical conditions, then it will have a higher priority than something only identified once. Notify the service development needs you have identified to those responsible for agreeing and implementing the development plans of the trust and/or practice.

Look back at your aspirations and standards set out in Stages 1 and 2. Match your learning or service development needs with one or more of these standards, or others that you have set yourself.

Stage 4: Make and carry out a learning and action plan with a timetable for your personal and service development

If you have not identified any learning needs for yourself or the service as a whole, you should omit Stage 4 and tidy up the presentation of your evidence for inclusion in your portfolio as at the end of Stage 5.

Think about whether:

- you have defined your learning objectives – what you need to learn to be able to attain the standards and outcomes you have described in Stage 2
- you can justify spending time and effort on the topics you prioritised in Stage 3. Is the topic important enough to your work, the NHS as a whole or patient safety? Does the clinical or non-clinical event occur sufficiently often to warrant the time spent?
- the time and resources for learning about that topic or making the associated changes to service delivery are available. Check that you are not trying to do too much too quickly, or you will become discouraged
- learning about that topic will make a difference to the care you or others can provide for patients
- and how one topic fits in with other topics you have identified to learn more about. Have you achieved a good balance across your areas of work or between your personal aspirations and the basic requirements of the service?

Decide on what method of learning is most appropriate for your task or role or the standards you are expecting to attain or sustain. You may have already identified your preferred learning style – but read up on this elsewhere if you are unsure.[7]

Describe how you will carry out your learning tasks and what you will do by a specified time. State how your learning will be applied and how and when it will be evaluated. Build in some staging posts so that you do not suddenly get to the end of 12 months and discover that you have only done half of your plan.

Your action plan should also include your role in remedying any gaps in service delivery that you identified in Stage 3 and that are within the remit of your responsibility.

Stage 5: Document your learning, competence, performance and standards of service delivery

You might choose to document that you have attained your defined outcomes by repeating the learning needs assessment that you started with. You could record your increased confidence and competence in dealing with situations that you previously avoided or performed inadequately.

You might incorporate your assessment of what has been gained in a study of another area that overlaps.

Preparing your portfolio[8–10]

Use your portfolio of evidence of what you have learnt and your standards of practice to:

- identify significant experiences to serve as important sources of learning
- reflect on the learning that arose from those experiences
- demonstrate learning in practice
- analyse and identify further learning needs and ways in which these needs can be met.

Your documentation might include all sorts of things, not just formal audits – although they make a good start. It might include reports of educational activities attended, statements of your roles and responsibilities, copies of publications you have read and critically appraised, and reports of your work. You could incorporate observations by others, evaluations of you observing other colleagues and how their practice differs from yours, descriptions of self-improvements, a video of typical activity, materials that demonstrate your skills to others, products of your input or learning – a new protocol for example. Box 1.3 gives a list of material you might include in your portfolio.

Box 1.3:   Possible contents of a portfolio
- Workload logs
- Case descriptions
- Videos
- Audiotapes
- Patient satisfaction surveys
- Research surveys
- Report of change or innovation
- Commentaries on published literature or books
- Records of critical incidents and learning points
- Notes from formal teaching sessions with reference to clinical work or other evidence

---

Once you are preparing to submit the portfolio for a discussion with a colleague (for example, at an appraisal) or assessment (for example, for a university postgraduate award or revalidation) write a self-assessment of your previous action plan. You might integrate your self-assessment into your PDP to show what you have achieved and what gaps you have still to address. Decide where are you now and where you want to be in one, three or five years' time. Select items from your portfolio for inclusion for each part of the documentation – you might have one compartment of your portfolio per speciality topic or section heading from *Good Medical Practice*.[3]

Make sure all references are included and the documentation in your portfolio is as accurate and complete as possible. Organise how you have shown your learning steps and your standards of practice so that it is indexed and cross-referenced to the relevant sections of the paperwork. Discuss the contents of your portfolio with a colleague or a mentor to gain other people's perspectives of your work and look for blind spots.

Include evidence of your competence as a GP with a special interest (GPwSI)

You may have a particular expertise or special interest in a clinical field or non-clinical area such as management, teaching or research. It may be that you have a lead role or responsibility in your practice for chronic disease management of clinical conditions such as diabetes, asthma, mental health or coronary heart disease. Or you may be employed by a PCO or hospital trust as a GPwSI to:

- lead in the development of services
- deliver a procedure-based service
- deliver an opinion-based service.

There is little consistency in extent of training or qualifications at present within or across the various GPwSI speciality areas.[11] Whatever your role or responsibility or expertise, your portfolio should include examples of evidence that show that you are competent, and that you have a consistently good performance in your speciality area. You may have parallel appraisals that you can include from your employer – for example, the university if you have a research or teaching post, or a hospital consultant if he or she supervises you in the clinical speciality.

When you gather evidence of your performance at work, try to document as many aspects of your work at one time as you can, so that for example an audit covers as many of the key headings from *Good Medical Practice* (*see* Box 1.1, page 5) as possible.[3] When you are identifying what you need to learn, or gaps in service delivery, make sure that you involve patients and show how you interact with the team. This gives you evidence about 'relationships with patients' and 'working with colleagues' as well as the clinical area you are focusing on or auditing.

Link your cycles of evidence to service developments rewarded by the new General Medical Services (GMS) Contract or Personal Medical Services (PMS) arrangements

The areas within the quality framework will probably be the ones that you prioritise in your PDP when looking at your service development needs.[12] The four main components of the quality framework are all relevant to your personal and professional development. The clinical and organisational standards may be those that you are aiming for in Stage 2 of the evidence cycle (*see* Figure 1.1). Achieving the standards in the quality framework will follow on from the descriptions of an excellent GP (Stage 1). Identifying personal learning needs and service development needs, that is, the gaps between baseline and specified standards in the quality framework, is in Stage 3. Making and carrying out your personal learning plan and service improvements in line with patients' experience is in Stage 4. Producing the documentation that shows you have attained the clinical or organisational standards required for core or additional services and responded to patients' views is in Stage 5.

References

1   Wakley G, Chambers R and Field S (2000) *Continuing Professional Development in Primary Care.* Radcliffe Medical Press, Oxford.

2   Royal College of General Practitioners/General Practitioners' Committee (2002) *Good Medical Practice for General Practitioners.* Royal College of General Practitioners, London.

3   General Medical Council (2001) *Good Medical Practice.* General Medical Council, London.

4   Department of Health (1998) *A First Class Service.* Department of Health, London.

5   Department of Health (1999) *Supporting Doctors, Protecting Patients.* Department of Health, London.

6   General Medical Council (2003) *Licence to Practise and Revalidation for Doctors.* General Medical Council, London. www.revalidationuk.info.

7   Mohanna K, Wall D and Chambers R (2003) *Teaching Made Easy: a manual for health professionals* (2e). Radcliffe Medical Press, Oxford.

8   Royal College of General Practitioners (1993) *Portfolio-based Learning in General Practice.* Occasional Paper 63, Royal College of General Practitioners, London.

9   Challis M (1999) AMEE Medical education guide No 11 (revised): portfolio-based learning and assessment in medical education. *Medical Teacher.* **21(4)**: 370–86.

10 Chambers R, Wakley G, Field S and Ellis S (2003) *Appraisal for the Apprehensive.* Radcliffe Medical Press, Oxford.

11 www.gpwsi.org.

12 General Practitioners' Committee/The NHS Confederation (2003) *New GMS Contract. Investing in general practice.* General Practitioners' Committee/NHS Confederation, London.

2

Practical ways to identify your learning and service needs as part of the documentation of your competence and performance

Setting standards to show that you are competent

Doctors 'must be committed to lifelong learning and be responsible for maintaining the medical knowledge and clinical and team skills necessary for the provision of quality care'.[1]

You could make a good start by describing your roles and responsibilities. This will help you to define what your competence should be now, or what competence you are hoping to attain (for instance as a GPwSI). Once you have your definition, you can recognise whether you have, or lack in some part, the necessary competence. If there are no accepted descriptions of competence in the area you are focusing on, then you will have to start from scratch. You might compile your description from national guidelines such as in the National Service Frameworks or health strategies. Usually you can find guidance about competency from specialist sources such as primary care associations for clinical topics or the various Royal Colleges. The Department of Health in England has worked with the Royal College of General Practitioners (RCGP) to describe the competency of GPs with special clinical interests in many clinical areas.[2]

A good definition of competence is someone who is: 'able to perform the tasks and roles required to the expected standard'.[3]

You will need to describe the standards expected in the range of tasks and roles you undertake and reference the source of standard setting. If professionals, or their organisations, are the only people involved in setting those standards, consider whether you should amend or extend the standards, tasks or roles by considering other perspectives such as those of patients or the NHS as a whole.

There is a difference between being competent, and performing in a consistently competent manner. You need to be motivated to perform consistently well and enabled to do so with efficient systems and sufficient resources. You will require sufficient numbers of other competent doctors or staff and available infrastructure such as diagnostic and treatment resources.[4]

Choose methods in Stage 3 (*see* Chapter 1) to demonstrate your standards of performance and identify any learning needs that span different topic areas, to reduce duplication and maximise the usefulness of your learning. Collecting evidence of more than one aspect of your competence or performance cuts down the overall amount of work underpinning your PDP or included in your appraisal portfolio.

Use several methods to identify your learning needs and/or gaps in your service development or delivery, so that you validate the findings of one method by another. No one method will give you reliable information about the gaps in your knowledge, skills or attitudes or everyday service. Does what you think about your performance match with what others in the team or patients think of how you practise in your everyday work? It is particularly difficult to determine what it is you 'don't know you don't know' by yourself, yet it is vital that you identify and rectify those gaps. Other people may be able to tell you what you need to learn quite readily. Colleagues from different disciplines could usefully comment on any shortfalls in how your work interfaces with theirs.

Patients or people who don't use your services could tell you whether the way you operate or provide services is off-putting or inappropriate. There may be data about your performance or that of your practice that could point out those gaps in your knowledge or skills of which you were previously unaware.

Determine what it is that you 'don't know you don't know' by:

- asking patients, users and non-users of your service
- comparing your performance against best practice or that of peers
- comparing your performance against objectives in business plans or national directives
- asking colleagues from different disciplines about shortfalls in how your work interfaces with theirs.

Identify your learning needs – how you can find out if you need to be better at doing your job

You may decide to use a few selected methods to gather baseline evidence of your performance, focused on your specific area of expertise. You may target other topics or areas at the same time that are relevant to the various sections of the GMC's booklet *Good Medical Practice*.[5] For this type of combined assessment, you might use several of the methods described in this chapter such as:

- constructive feedback from peers or patients
- 360° feedback
- self-assessment, or review by others, using a rating scale to assess your skills and attitudes
- comparison with protocols and guidelines for checking how well procedures are followed
- audit: various types and applications
- significant event audit
- eliciting patient views such as in satisfaction surveys
- a SWOT (strengths, weaknesses, opportunities and threats) or SCOT (strengths, challenges, opportunities and threats) analysis
- reading and reflecting
- educational review.

Several of these methods will also be useful for identifying service development needs – you can look at the gaps identified from both the personal and service perspectives at the same time using the same method.

Seek feedback

Find colleagues who will give you constructive feedback about your performance and practice. The golden rule for giving constructive feedback is to give positive praise of things that have been well done first. Sometimes colleagues launch straight in to criticise faults when asked for their views. The Pendleton model of the giving of feedback is widely used in the health setting (*see* Box 2.1).[6]

Box 2.1: The Pendleton model of giving feedback[6]

1 The 'learner' goes first and performs the activity.
2 Questions clarify any facts.
3 The 'learner' says what they thought was done well.
4 The 'teacher' says what they thought was done well.
5 The 'learner' says what could be improved upon.
6 The 'teacher' says what could be improved upon.
7 Both discuss ideas for improvements in a helpful and constructive manner.

360° feedback

This collects together perceptions from a number of different participants as shown in Figure 2.1.

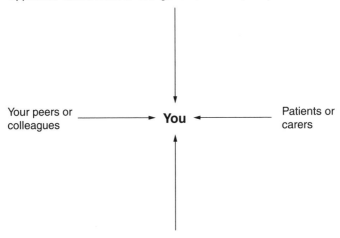

People to whom you are responsible: managers in your PCO, appraiser, clinical lead, clinical governance lead, GP partners etc.

Your peers or colleagues ⟶ **You** ⟵ Patients or carers

People responsible to you: clinical and non-clinical staff

Figure 2.1:   360° feedback.

The wider the spread of people giving feedback, the more rounded the picture. Each individual gives a feedback questionnaire to at least three people in each of the groups above. An independent person then collects and collates the questionnaires and discusses the results with the individual. Computerised versions are available from commercial companies.[7] The main disadvantage of this method is that it can sometimes be spoilt by malicious comments against which individuals cannot readily defend themselves.

Self-assess or gain another person's perspective on your standard of practice or service delivery

You might describe any aspect of your practice as statements (A to G as in Box 2.2) about your competence or performance for you to self-assess, or others to give you feedback or comments by marking the extent to which they agree on the linear scales opposite. You could use the descriptions of an excellent GP in *Good Medical Practice for General Practitioners*[8] as we have done in relating statements in Box 2.2 to consultation skills. For instance, if statement A is: 'I consistently treat patients politely and with consideration',[8] you could self-assess the extent to which you agree. Alternatively, you could ask colleagues or patients to fill in the assessment form. Objective feedback from external assessment is usually more reliable than your own self-assessment when you may have blind spots about your own performance. As you become more confident in this method of reviewing your competence, you might emphasise how consistent you are in your application of good practice – so in the statements below we have sometimes included 'consistently', 'always' or 'usually'. You can set your own challenges. If you have a mentor or a 'buddy' in the practice with whom you learn, you might discuss and reflect on the completed marking grids with him or her.

Box 2.2: Marking grid: circle the number which represents your views or feelings about each statement – complete the grid on more than one occasion and compare results over time

A   I consistently treat patients politely and with consideration.
STRONGLY AGREE   to   STRONGLY DISAGREE

1-----------------2-----------------3-----------------4-----------------5-----------------6

B   I am aware of how my personal beliefs could affect the care offered to the patient, and take care not to impose my own beliefs and values.
STRONGLY AGREE   to   STRONGLY DISAGREE

1-----------------2-----------------3-----------------4-----------------5-----------------6

C   I always treat all patients equally and ensure that some groups are not favoured at the expense of others.
STRONGLY AGREE   to   STRONGLY DISAGREE

1-----------------2-----------------3-----------------4-----------------5-----------------6

D   I try to maintain a relationship with the patient or family when a mistake has occurred.
STRONGLY AGREE   to   STRONGLY DISAGREE

1-----------------2-----------------3-----------------4-----------------5-----------------6

E   I always obtain informed consent to treatment.
STRONGLY AGREE   to   STRONGLY DISAGREE

1-----------------2-----------------3-----------------4-----------------5-----------------6

F   I usually involve patients in decisions about their care.
STRONGLY AGREE   to   STRONGLY DISAGREE

1-----------------2-----------------3-----------------4-----------------5-----------------6

G   I always respect the right of patients to refuse treatments or tests.
STRONGLY AGREE   to   STRONGLY DISAGREE

1-----------------2-----------------3-----------------4-----------------5-----------------6

Compare your performance against protocols or guidelines

Are you familiar with all the protocols or guidelines that are used by someone, somewhere in the practice? You might determine your learning needs and those of other practice team members by piling all the protocols or guidelines that exist in your practice in a big heap and rationalising them so that you have a common set across the practice. Working as a team you can compare your own knowledge and usual practice with others and with protocols or guidelines recommended by the National Institute for Clinical Excellence (NICE)[9] or National Service Frameworks or the Scottish Intercollegiate Guidelines Network (SIGN).[10]

Alternatively, you might compare your own practice against a protocol or guideline that is generally accepted at a national or local level. You could audit the standard of your practice to find out how often you adhere to such a protocol or guideline, and if you can justify why you deviate from the recommendations.

Audit

Audit is:

> the method used by health professionals to assess, evaluate, and improve the care of patients in a systematic way, to enhance their health and quality of life.[11]

The five steps of the audit cycle are shown in Box 2.3.

Box 2.3:   The five steps of the audit cycle

1   Describe the criteria and standards you are trying to achieve.
2   Measure your current performance of how well you are providing care or services in an objective way.
3   Compare your performance against criteria and standards.
4   Identify the need for change – to performance, adjustment of criteria or standards, resources, available data.
5   Make any required changes as necessary and re-audit later.

Performance or practice is often broken down for the purposes of audit into the three aspects of structure, process and outcome. Structural audits might concern resources such as equipment, premises, skills, people, etc. Process audits focus on what is done to the patient: for instance, clinical protocols and guidelines. Audits of outcomes consider the impact of care or services on the patient and might include patient satisfaction, health gains and effectiveness of care or services. You might look at aspects of quality of the structure, process and outcome of the delivery of any clinical field, focusing on access, equity of care between different groups in the population, efficiency, economy, effectiveness for individual patients, etc.[11]

Set standards for your performance, find out how you are doing, search to find out best practice, make the changes and then re-audit the care given to patients in the future with the same problem. Some variations on audit include:

- *Case note analysis.* This gives an insight into your current practice. It might be a retrospective review of a random selection of notes, or a prospective survey of consecutive patients with the same condition as they present to see you.
- *Peer review.* Compare an area of practice with other individual professionals or managers; or compare practice teams as a whole. An independent body might compare all practices in one area e.g. within a primary care trust (PCT) or organisation so that like is compared with like. Feedback may be arranged to protect participants' identities so that only the individual person or practice knows their own identity, the rest being anonymised, for example by giving each practice a number. Where there is mutual trust and an open learning culture, peer review does not need to be anonymised and everyone can learn together about making improvements in practice.
- *Criteria based audit.* This compares clinical practice with specific standards, guidelines or protocols. Re-audit of changes should demonstrate improvements in the quality of patient care.
- *External audit.* Prescribing advisers or managers in PCOs can supply information about indicators of performance for audit. Visits from external bodies such as the Commission for Healthcare Audit and Inspection (CHAI) expose the PCO or hospital trust in England and Wales to external audit.
- *Tracer criteria.* Assessing the quality of care of a 'tracer' condition may be used to represent the quality of care of other similar conditions or more complex problems. Tracer criteria should be easily defined and measured. For instance, if you were to audit the extent to which you reviewed repeat prescriptions, you might focus on a drug such as thyroxine and generalise from your audit results to your likely performance with other medications.

Significant event audit

Think of an incident where a patient or you experienced an adverse event. This might be an unexpected death, an unplanned pregnancy, an avoidable side-effect from prescribed medication, a violent attack on a member of staff, or an angry outburst in public by you or a work colleague. You can review the case and reflect on the sequence of events that led to that critical event occurring. It is likely that there were a multitude of factors leading up to that significant event. You should take the case to a multidisciplinary meeting to reflect and analyse what were the triggers, causes and consequences of the event. Complete the significant event audit cycle by planning what individuals, or the practice as a whole, might do to avoid a similar event happening in future. This might include undertaking further learning and/or making appropriate changes to the practice or your systems.

The steps of a significant event audit are shown in Box 2.4.

Box 2.4: Steps of a significant event audit

- *Step 1*: Describe who was involved, what time of day, what the task/activity was, the context and any other relevant information.
- *Step 2*: Reflect on the effects of the event on the participants and the professionals involved.
- *Step 3*: Discuss the reasons for the event or situation arising with other colleagues, review case notes or other records.
- *Step 4*: Decide how you or others might have behaved differently. Describe your options for how the procedures at work might be changed to minimise or eliminate chances of the event recurring.
- *Step 5*: Plan changes that are needed, how they will be implemented, who will be responsible for what and when, what further training or resources are required. Then carry out the changes.
- *Step 6*: Re-audit later to see whether changes to procedures or new knowledge and skills are having the desired effects. Give feedback to the practice team.

An assessment by an external body

This is a traditional way of showing that you are competent by taking and passing an examination. It is a good way of testing recalled knowledge in a written or oral examination, or establishing how you behave in a clinical situation on the day of a practical examination, but not much good for measuring anything else. A summative examination (i.e. done at the end of a course of study) gives a measure of your learning up to that date.

You might undertake an objective test of your knowledge and skills. Examples are a computer-based test in the form of multiple-choice questions and patient management problems as in the RCGP's phased evaluation programme (PEP) CD ROMs (email pep@rcgp-scotland.org.uk) or the Apollo programme available from BMJ Publishing.[12] Various other organisations give multiple-choice question-naires that you can complete on paper or online and record in your portfolio.[13,14]

The RCGP's series of quality awards provide external assessment – Membership by Assessment of Performance, Fellowship by Assessment, Quality Team Development, etc. Trained assessors will give feedback to individual doctors or practice teams about their performance compared with set standards and their peers.

Elicit the views of patients

Part of meeting the criteria for relationships with patients in *Good Medical Practice*[5] might be to assess patients' satisfaction with:

- you
- your practice
- the local hospital's way of working
- other services available in your locality.

Avoid surveys where questions are relatively superficial or biased. A more specific enquiry should uncover particular elements of patients' dissatisfaction, which will be more useful if you are trying to identify your learning needs. Use a well-validated patient questionnaire such as the General Practice Assessment Questionnaire (GPAQ)[15] or the Doctors' Interpersonal Skills Questionnaire (DISQ)[16] instead of risking producing your own version with ambiguities and flaws. Many doctors and practice teams have used these patient survey methods, providing a bank of data against which to compare your performance.

Other sources of feedback from patients might be obtained through suggestion boxes for patients to contribute comments, or the practice team recording all patients' suggestions and complaints however trivial, looking for patterns in the comments received.

There will be learning to be had from every complaint – even if the complaint does not have any substance, there should be something to learn about the shortfall in communication between you and the complainant.

The evolving of the 'expert patient programme' should mean that there is a pool of well informed patients with chronic conditions who can contribute their insights into what you (or the service) need to learn from a patient's perspective.[17]

Strengths, weaknesses (or challenges), opportunities and threats (SWOT or SCOT) analysis

You can undertake a SWOT (or SCOT) analysis of your own performance or that of your practice team or practice organisation, working it out on your own, or with a workmate or mentor, or with a group of colleagues. Brainstorm the strengths, weaknesses (or challenges), opportunities and threats of your role or circumstances.

Strengths and weaknesses (or challenges) of your roles might relate to your clinical knowledge or skills, experience, expertise, decision making, communication skills, interprofessional relationships, political skills, timekeeping, organisational skills, teaching skills, or research skills. Strengths and weaknesses (or challenges) of the practice organisation might relate to most of these aspects as well as the way resources are allocated, overall efficiency and the degree to which the practice is patient centred.

Opportunities might relate to your unexploited experience or potential strengths, expected changes in the NHS, or resources for which you might bid. For example, you might train for and set up a special interest post.

Threats will include factors and circumstances that prevent you from achieving your aims for personal, professional and practice development or service improvements. They might be to do with your health, turnover in the practice team, or time-limited investment by the PCO.

List the important factors in your SWOT (or SCOT) analysis in order of priority through discussion with colleagues and independent people from outside your practice. Draw up goals and a timed action plan for you or the practice team to follow.

Informal conversations – in the corridor, over coffee

You learn such a lot when chatting with colleagues at coffee time or over a meal and can become aware of your learning or service development needs at these times. This is when you realise that other people are doing things differently from you and if they seem to be doing it better and achieving more, you can challenge yourself to decide if this matter could be one of your blind spots. Note down your thoughts before you forget them so that you can reflect on them later.

Online discussion groups may provide another source of informal exchanges with colleagues. If you find this difficult to start with, you might 'lurk', viewing the comments and views of other people until you feel confident enough to contribute. Record any observations that you find useful and reflect on how they might inform your own practice.

Observe your work environment and role

Observation could be informal and opportunistic, or more systematic, working through a structured checklist. One method of self-assessment might be to audiotape yourself at work dealing with patients (after obtaining patients' informed consent). Listen to the tape afterwards to appraise your communication and consultation skills – on your own or with a friend or colleague. If you have access to video equipment, you might use this instead.

Look at the equipment in your practice or your emergency bag. Do you know how to operate it properly? Assess yourself undertaking practical procedures or ask someone to watch you operate the equipment or undertaking the practical procedure and give you feedback about your performance.

Analyse the various roles and responsibilities of your current posts. Compare your level of expertise against national standards such as in the Knowledge and Skills Framework for England from the Department of Health or a job evaluation framework as part of the Agenda for Change initiative.[18,19] Determine if you can meet the requirements, or, if not, what deficiencies need to be made good.

You might combine one of the methods of identifying your learning needs already described such as an audit or SWOT analysis and apply it to 'observing your work environment or role', describing your relationship with other members of the multidisciplinary team for example, or reviewing how their roles and responsibilities interface with yours.

Read and reflect

When reading articles in respected journals, reflect on what the key messages mean for you in your situation. Note down topics about which you know little but that are relevant to your work, and calculate if you have further learning needs not met by the article you are reading. If the article is relevant to your practice, record what changes you will make and how you will make the changes. Record how you will impart your new knowledge to others in your practice.

Educational review

You might find a 'buddy' or work colleague, CPD tutor, or a clinical tutor or clinical supervisor with whom you can have an informal or formal discussion about your performance, job situation and learning needs. You might draw up a learning contract as a result with a timed plan of action.

Identify your service needs – how you can find out if there are gaps in services or how you deliver care

Now focus your attention on the needs of your practice or the PCO. The standards of service delivery should be those that allow you to practise as a competent clinician. You may be competent but be unable to perform or practice to a competent level if the resources available to you are inadequate, or other colleagues have insufficient knowledge or skills to support you. You cannot be expected to take responsibility for ensuring that resources you need to be able to practise in a competent manner are available. However, as a professional you should play a significant role in collecting evidence to make a case for the need for essential resources to your GP colleagues, the practice manager, staff at the trust or PCO or whoever is appropriate.

Some of the methods you might use are described below and include:

- involving patients and the public in giving you feedback about the quality and quantity of your services
- monitoring access and availability to care
- undertaking a force-field analysis
- assessing risk
- evaluating the standards of care or services you provide
- comparing the systems in your practice with those required by legislation
- considering your patient population's health needs
- reviewing teamwork
- assessing the quality of your services
- reflecting on whether you are providing cost-effective care and services.

Involve patients and the public in giving you feedback about the quality and quantity of your services

Patient and public involvement may occur at three levels:

1   for individual patients about their own care
2   for patients and the public about the range and quality of health services on offer
3   in planning and organising health service developments.

The phrase 'patient and public involvement' is used here to mean individual involvement as a user, patient or carer; or public involvement that includes the processes of consultation and participation.[20]

If a patient involvement or public consultation exercise is to be meaningful, it has to involve people who represent the section of the population that the exercise is about. You will have to set up systems to actively seek out and involve people from minority groups or those with sensory impairments such as blind and deaf people.

Before you start:

- define the purpose
- be realistic about the magnitude of the planned exercise
- select an appropriate method or several methods depending on the target population and your resources
- obtain the commitment of everyone who will be affected by the exercise
- frame the method in accordance with your perspective
- write the protocol.

You might hold focus groups, or set up a patient panel, or invite feedback and help from a patient participation group. You could interview patients selected either at random from the patient population or for their experience of a particular condition or circumstance.

Monitor access and availability to healthcare

Access and availability

You could look at waiting times to see a health professional by using:

- computerised appointment lists or paper and pen to record the time of arrival, the time of the appointment, the time seen
- the next available appointments that can easily be monitored by computer, or more painfully by manual searches of the appointment books.

Compare the results at intervals (a spreadsheet is a good way to do this). Do you or your staff have learning needs in relation to the use of technology, or new ways of redesigning the service you offer?

Referrals to other agencies and hospitals

You might audit and re-audit the time taken from the date the patient is seen to:

- the referral being sent (do you need more secretarial time?)
- the date the patient is seen by the other agency (could the patient be seen elsewhere quicker or do you need to liaise with other agencies over referrals?)
- the date the patient's needs have been met by investigation, diagnosis, treatment, provision of aid or support, etc. (can you influence how quickly these are completed?).

Identify any learning needs here. For instance, new methods of teamwork with a different mix of skills between doctors, nurses and non-clinically qualified assistants could provide extra services in the practice, or you, or a colleague, might retrain to become a GP with a special clinical interest.

Draw up a force-field analysis

This tool will help you to identify and focus down on the positive and negative forces in your work and to gain an overview of the weighting of these factors. Draw a horizontal or vertical line in the middle of a sheet of paper. Label one side 'positive' and the other side 'negative'. Draw bars to represent individual positive drivers that motivate you on one side of the line, and factors that are demotivating on the other negative side of the line. The thickness and length of the bars should represent the extent of the influence; that is, a short, narrow bar will indicate that the positive or negative factor has a minor influence and a long, wide bar a major effect. *See* Box 2.5 for an example.

Box 2.5:   Example of force-field analysis diagram. Satisfaction with current post as a health professional

Positive factors (driving forces)	Negative factors (restraining forces)
career aspirations	long hours of work
salary	demands from patients
autonomy	
satisfaction from caring	job insecurity
no uniform	oppressive hierarchy
opportunities for professional development	

Take an overview of the resulting force-field diagram and consider if you are content with things as they are, or can think of ways to boost the positive side and minimise the negative factors. You can do this part of the exercise on your own, with a peer or a small group in the practice, or with a mentor or someone from outside the practice. The exercise should help you to realise the extent to which a known influence in your life, or in the practice as a whole, is a positive or negative factor. Make a personal or organisational action plan to create the situations and opportunities to boost the positive factors in your life and minimise the bars on the negative side.

Assess risk

Risk assessment might entail evaluating the risks to the health or well-being or competence of yourself, staff and/or patients in your practice or workplace, and deciding on the action needed to minimise or eliminate those risks.[21]

- *A hazard*: something with the potential to cause harm.
- *A risk*: the likelihood of that potential to cause harm being realised.

There are five steps to risk assessment:

1 look for and list the hazards
2 decide who might be harmed and how
3 evaluate the risks arising from the hazards and decide whether existing precautions are adequate or more should be done
4 record the findings
5 review your assessment from time to time and revise it if necessary.

You do not want to spend a lot of time and effort identifying risks or making changes if they do not matter much. When you have identified a risk, consider:

- is the risk large?
- does it happen often?
- is it a significant risk?

Risks may be prevented, avoided, minimised or managed where they cannot be eliminated. You, your colleagues and your staff may need to learn how to do this.

Record significant events where someone has experienced an adverse event or had a near miss – as part of you identifying your service development needs on an ongoing basis. Most significant incidents do not have one cause. Usually there are faults in the system, which are compounded by someone or several people being careless, tired, overworked or ill-informed. Cultivate an atmosphere of openness and discussion without blame so that you can all learn from the significant event. If people think they will be blamed they will hide the incident and no one will be able to prevent it happening again. Look for *all* the causes and try to remedy as many as possible to prevent the situation from arising in the future.

Evaluate the standards of services or care you provide

Keep your evaluation as simple as possible. Avoid wasting resources on unnecessarily bureaucratic evaluation. Design the evaluation so that you:

- specify the event (such as a service) to be evaluated – define broad issues, set priorities against strategic goals, time and resources, seek agreement on the nature and scope of the task
- describe the expected impact of the programme or activity and who will be affected
- define the criteria of success – these might relate to structure, process or outcome
- identify the information required to demonstrate the achievements of the programme or activity. The record might include: observing behaviour; data from existing records; prospective recording by the subjects of the programme or by the recipients and staff of the activity
- determine the time frame for the evaluation
- specify who collects the data for all stages in the delivery of the programme or activity, and the respective deadlines
- review and refine the objectives of the programme or activity and check that they are appropriate for the outcomes and impact you expect.

What to evaluate?

You could:

- adopt any, or all, of the six aspects of the health service's performance assessment framework (*see* Box 2.6)
- agree milestones and goals at stages in your programme or adopt others such as those relating to the National Service Frameworks for coronary heart disease or mental health
- evaluate the extent to which you achieve the outcome(s) starting with an objective. Alternatively, you might evaluate how conducive is the context of the programme, or activity, to achieving the anticipated outcomes
- undertake regular audits of aspects of the structure, process and outcome of a service or project to see if you have achieved what you expected when you established the criteria and standards of the audit programme
- evaluate the various components of a new system or programme: the activities, personnel involved, provision of services, organisational structure, precise goals and interventions.

Box 2.6: The six aspects of the NHS performance assessment framework

1 Health improvement
2 Fair access
3 Effective delivery
4 Efficiency
5 Patient/carer experience
6 Health outcomes

Computer search

The extent to which you can evaluate your practice will depend on the quality of your records and extent to which you use the capacity of your practice computer. Compare the results of a computerised search for all those using one type of treatment with another. Make appropriate changes to your systems depending on what the computer search reveals. Put your plan into action and monitor with repeat searches at regular intervals.

Look at your learning or service development needs by analysing data from practice records to:

- look at trends and patterns of illness
- devise and use clinical guidelines and decision support systems as part of evidence-based practice
- audit what you are doing
- provide the information on which to base decisions on commissioning and management
- support epidemiology, research and teaching activities.

Compare the systems in your practice with those required by legislation

Legislation changes quite frequently. As an employer, a GP needs to keep abreast of the legislation or ensure that the practice manager does so. You could start by comparing the systems in your practice with those required by the Disability Discrimination Act (1995) and health and safety legislation.

Consider your patient population's health needs

Create a detailed profile of your practice population. Ask your PCO or public health lead for information about your practice population and comparative information about the general population living in the district – morbidity and mortality statistics, referral patterns, age/sex mix, ethnicity, and population trends.

   Include information about the wider determinants of health such as housing, numbers of the population in, and types of, employment, geographical location, the environment, crime and safety, educational attainment and socio-economic data. Make a note of any particular health problems such as higher than average teenage pregnancy rates or drug misuse. Focus on the current state of health inequalities within your practice population or between your practice population and the district as a whole. It may be that circumstances change, which in turn alters the proportion of minority groups in your practice population – such as if a continuing care home opens up in your practice area, or there is an influx of homeless people or asylum seekers into your locality.

Review teamwork

You can measure how effective the team is[22] – evaluate whether the team has:

- clear goals and objectives
- accountability and authority
- individual roles for members
- shared tasks
- regular internal formal and informal communication
- full participation by members
- confrontation of conflict
- feedback to individuals
- feedback about team performance
- outside recognition
- two-way external communication
- team rewards.

Assess the quality of your services

Quality may be subdivided into eight components: equity, access, acceptability and responsiveness, appropriateness, communication, continuity, effectiveness and efficiency.[23]

   You might use the matrix in Box 2.7 as a way of ordering your approach to auditing a particular topic with the eight aspects of quality on the vertical axis, and structure, process and outcome on the horizontal axis.[24] In this way you can generate up to 24 aspects of a particular topic. You might then focus on several aspects to look at the quality of patient care or services from various angles.

Box 2.7:   Matrix for assessing the quality of a clinical service

You might like to look at the structure, process or outcome of communicating test results to patients, for example:

	Structure	Process	Outcome
Equity			
Access			
Acceptability and responsiveness			
Appropriateness			
Communication	Hospital report	Feedback	Action taken
Effectiveness			
Efficiency			

Look for service development needs reflecting why patients receive a poor quality of service such as:

- inadequately trained staff or staff with poor levels of competence
- lack of confidentiality
- staff not being trained in the management of emergency situations
- doctors or nurses not being contactable in an emergency or being ineffective
- treatment being unavailable due to poor management of resources or services
- poor management of the arrangements for home visiting
- insufficient numbers of available staff for the workload
- qualifications of locums or deputising staff being unknown or inadequate for the posts they are filling
- arrangements for transfer of information from one team member to another being inadequate
- team members not acting on information received.

Many of these items will need action as a team, but for some of them, it may be your responsibility to ensure that adequate standards are met.

Reflect on whether you are providing cost-effective care and services

Cost-effectiveness is not synonymous with 'cheap'. A cost-effective intervention is one which gives a better or equivalent benefit from the intervention in question for lower or equivalent cost, or where the relative improvement in outcome is higher than the relative difference in cost. In other words being cost-effective means having the best outcomes for the least input. Using the term 'cost-effective' implies that you have considered potential alternatives.

An intervention must first be considered *clinically* effective to warrant investigation into its potential to be *cost*-effective. Evidence-based practice must incorporate clinical judgement. You have to interpret the evidence when it comes to applying it to individual patients, whether it is evidence about clinical effectiveness or cost-effectiveness. A new or alternative treatment or intervention should be compared directly with the previous best treatment or intervention.

An economic evaluation is a comparative analysis of two or more alternatives in terms of their costs and consequences. There are four different types as shown in Box 2.8.

Box 2.8:   The four types of economic evaluation

1   *Cost-effectiveness analysis* is used to compare the effectiveness of two interventions with the same treatment objectives.
2   *Cost minimisation* compares the costs of alternative treatments that have identical health outcomes.
3   *Cost–utility analysis* enables the effects of alternative interventions to be measured against a combination of life expectancy and quality of life; common outcome measures are quality adjusted life years (QALYs) or health-related quality of life (hrqol).
4   *Cost–benefit analysis* is a technique designed to determine the feasibility of a project, plan, management or treatment by quantifying its costs and benefits. It is often difficult to determine these accurately in relation to health.

While health valuation is unavoidable, it cannot be objective. You will probably have learning needs around what subjective method is best to use.[25]

Efficiency is sometimes confused with effectiveness. Being efficient means obtaining the most quality from the least expenditure, or the required level of quality for the least expenditure. To measure efficiency you need to make a judgement about the level of quality of the 'purchase' and be able to relate it to 'price'. 'Price' alone does not measure efficiency. Quality is the indicator used in combination with price to assess if something is more efficient. So, cost-effectiveness is a measure of efficiency and suggests that costs have been related to effectiveness.

Consider if you have service development needs. Discuss whether:

- the current skill mix in your team is appropriate
- more cost-effective alternative types of delivery of care are available
- sufficient staff training exists for those taking on new roles and responsibilities.

Set priorities: how you match what's needed with what's possible

You and your colleagues will have been able to make a wish list after following the previous Stage 3 undertaking a variety of needs assessments. Group and summarise your learning and service development needs from the exercises you have carried out. Grade them according to the priority you set. You may put one at a higher priority because it fits in with learning needs established from another section, or put another lower because it does not fit in with other activities that you will put into your learning plan for the next 12 months. If you have identified a learning need by several different methods of assessment then it will have a higher priority than something only identified once in your PDP. Collect information from all the team, the patients, users and carers to feed back before you make a decision on how to progress. Remember to consider external influences such as the National Service Frameworks, NICE guidance, governmental priorities, priorities of your PCO, the content of the Local Delivery Plan, etc.

Select those topics that are tied into organisational priorities, have clear aims and objectives and are achievable within your time and resource constraints. When ranking topics for learning or action in order of priority (Stage 4) consider whether:

- the project aims and objectives are clearly defined
- the topic is important:
  - for the population served (e.g. the size of the problem and/or its severity)
  - for the skills, knowledge or attitudes of the individual or team
- it is feasible
- it is affordable
- it will make enough difference
- it fits in with other priorities.

You will still have more ideas than can possibly be implemented. Remember the highest priority – the health service is for patients that use it or who will do so in the future.

References

1   Medical Professionalism Project (2002) Medical professionalism in the new millennium: a physicians' charter. *Lancet.* **359**: 520–2.

2   www.gpwsi.org/subindex.shtml.

3   Eraut M and du Boulay B (2000) *Developing the Attributes of Medical Professional Judgement and Competence.* University of Sussex, Sussex. Reproduced at www.cogs.susx.ac.uk/users/bend/doh.

4   Fraser SW and Greenhalgh T (2001) Coping with complexity: educating for capability. *British Medical Journal.* **323**: 799–802.

5   General Medical Council (2001) *Good Medical Practice.* General Medical Council, London.

6   Pendleton D, Schofield T, Tate P and Havelock P (2003) *The New Consultation, Developing Doctor–Patient Communication.* Oxford University Press, Oxford.

7   King J (2002) Career focus: 360° appraisal. *British Medical Journal.* **324**: S195.

8   Royal College of General Practitioners/General Practitioners' Committee (2002) *Good Medical Practice for General Practitioners.* Royal College of General Practitioners, London.

9   National Institute for Clinical Excellence (NICE) www.nice.org.uk.

10 Scottish Intercollegiate Guidelines Network (SIGN) www.sign.ac.uk.

11 Irvine D and Irvine S (eds) (1991) *Making Sense of Audit.* Radcliffe Medical Press, Oxford.

12 Toon P, Greenhalgh T, Rigby M *et al.* (2002) *The Human Face of Medicine.* Two CD ROMs in the APOLLO (Advancing Professional Practice through Online Learning Opportunities) series. BMJ Publishing Group, London. Free sample available at www.apollobmj.com.

13 *Guidelines in Practice* www.eguidelines.co.uk.

14 www.doctors.net.uk.

15 www.npcrdc.man.ac.uk.

16 http://www.ex.ac./cfep.

17 Department of Health (2003) *EPP Update Newsletter.* DoH, London. *See* Expert Patient Programme on www.ohn.gov.uk/ohn/people/expert.htm.

18 Department of Health (2003) *The NHS Knowledge and Skills Framework (NHS KSF) and Development Review Guidance – working draft.* Version 6. Department of Health, London.

19 Department of Health (2003) *Job Evaluation Handbook.* Version 1. Department of Health, London.

20 Chambers R, Drinkwater C and Boath E (2003) *Involving Patients and the Public: how to do it better* (2e). Radcliffe Medical Press, Oxford.

21 Mohanna K and Chambers R (2000) *Risk Matters in Healthcare.* Radcliffe Medical Press, Oxford.

22 Hart E and Fletcher J (1999) Learning how to change: a selective analysis of literature and experience of how teams learn and organisations change. *Journal of Interprofessional Care.* **13(1)**: 53–63.

23 Maxwell RJ (1984) Quality assessment in health. *British Medical Journal.* **288**: 1470–2.

24 Firth-Cozens J (1993) *Audit in Mental Health Services.* LEA, Hove.

25 McCulloch D (2003) *Valuing Health in Practice.* Ashgate Publishing Ltd, Aldershot.

3

Demonstrating common components of good quality healthcare

In looking at the quality of care you provide and demonstrating your standards of service delivery and outcomes of learning, you should find that obtaining informed consent from patients for their treatment, maintaining confidentiality and handling complaints are part of the fabric of good quality care. We have considered them separately in this chapter, but each may be individualised to any of the seven clinical areas of Chapters 4 to 10.

We have set out the chapter with key information about consent followed by some example cycles of the stages of evidence (see Figure 1.1 on page 6). The two other sections on confidentiality and complaints follow, laid out in similar ways. Read through the cycles of evidence to become familiar with the approach to gathering and documenting evidence of your learning, competence, performance or standards of service delivery. Then either adopt one of the examples or adapt it to your own circumstances. Alternatively, look at these three components in a clinical context in relation to other subjects as illustrated in the subsequent clinical chapters.

Consent

Key points

Information given to a health professional remains the property of the patient. In most circumstances, consent is assumed for the necessary sharing of information with other professionals involved with the care of the patient for that episode of care. Usually consent is also assumed for essential sharing of information for continuing care. Beyond this, informed consent must be obtained. Patients attend for healthcare in the belief that the personal information that they supply, or which is found out about them during investigation or treatment, will be confidential.

Exceptions to the above are:[1]

- if the patient consents
- if it is in the patient's own interest that information should be disclosed, but it is either impossible to seek the patient's consent or
- it is medically undesirable in the patient's own interest, to seek the patient's consent
- if the law requires (and does not merely permit) the health professional to disclose the information
- if the health professional has an overriding duty to society to disclose the information
- if the health professional agrees with a governmental agency that disclosure is necessary to safeguard national security
- if the disclosure is necessary to prevent a serious risk to public health
- in certain circumstances, for the purposes of medical research.

> Health professionals must be able to justify their decision to disclose information without consent. If they are in any doubt, they should consult their professional bodies and colleagues.

Consent is only valid if the patient fully understands the nature and consequences of disclosure – they must be able to give their consent, receive enough information to enable them to make a decision and be acting under their own free will and not persuaded by the strong influence of another person. If consent is given, the health worker is responsible for limiting the disclosure to that information for which informed consent has been obtained. The development of modern information technology and the increasing amount of multidisciplinary teamwork in patient care make confidentiality difficult to uphold.

You may need to give information about a patient to a relative or carer. Normally the consent of the patient should be obtained. Sometimes, the clinical condition of the patient may prevent informed consent being obtained (e.g. they are unconscious or have a severe illness). It is important to recognise that relatives or carers do not have any right to information about the patient. Disclosure without consent may be justified when third parties are exposed to a risk so serious that it outweighs the patient's privacy. An example would be if a patient declines to allow you to disclose information about their health and continues to drive against medical advice when unfit to do so.

Local research ethics committees and the research governance framework ensure best practice in the giving of informed consent by patients in research studies.

As health professionals, we often assume implied consent. The public and patients are generally ignorant of the extent to which information about them is passed around the NHS. When teaching at both undergraduate and postgraduate levels, in examinations and assessments and in research, we may incorrectly assume that patients imply their consent. Consent is also implied for health service accounting, central monitoring of referrals, in disease registers, for audit and in facilitating joint working between team members. The NHS is still engaged in a debate about what data can legitimately be shared without patients' explicit consent. Although written consent is usually obtained for supplying information to insurance companies or for legal reports, patients are often unaware of the type of information being supplied and have not given 'informed consent'. Guidelines published jointly by the British Medical Association (BMA) and the Association of British Insurers clarify that doctors are not required to release all aspects of a patient's medical history but need only submit (with the patient's consent) information that is relevant.[2]

The GMC's booklet *Seeking Patients' Consent: the ethical considerations* explores issues of consent in more depth and advises that

> the amount of information you give each patient will vary according to factors such as the nature of the condition, the complexity of the treatment, the risks associated with the treatment or procedure and the patient's own wishes ... you should be careful about relying on a patient's apparent compliance with a procedure as a form of consent.[3]

Consent to treatment with medication is often assumed[4–7] – the doctor prescribes the medication and the patient takes it. However, we know that a prescription may not be taken to the pharmacy for dispensing, or if it is, the medication may not be started, or continued. You need to think about how you can move from compliance to concordance as defined below.

- *Compliance* with treatment or lifestyle changes implies that the patient follows instructions from health professionals to a greater or lesser degree.
- *Concordance* is a negotiated agreement on treatment between the patient and the healthcare professional. It allows patients to take informed decisions on the degree of risk or suffering that they themselves wish to undertake or follow.

Collecting data to demonstrate your learning, competence, performance and standards of service delivery: consent

Example cycle of evidence 3.1

- Focus: informed consent
- Other relevant foci: relationships with patients; concordance

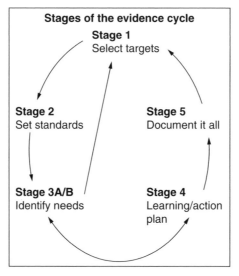

Stages of the evidence cycle

Stage 1
Select targets

Stage 2
Set standards

Stage 5
Document it all

Stage 3A/B
Identify needs

Stage 4
Learning/action plan

Box 3.1:   Case study

Mrs Humble comes into surgery to see you for a review of her medication. She is already on medication for her hypertension, but her last three readings by the practice nurse are still raised, her total cholesterol is 8 mmol/l and her body mass index (BMI) has increased to 38. You briefly go through the alternatives that are open to her as a 45-year-old smoker. Her eye contact is poor and, when you ask her what she thinks, she says 'Whatever you think best, doctor'. Looking at her medical record, it shows that she doesn't always remember to renew her prescription on time. When you ask about what time she takes her tablet and how she reminds herself to take them, she looks away and says that it's very difficult to remember everything. You ask about her diet and smoking and she looks even more dejected, saying that she will have to try again. You give her some written information about hypertension to read and arrange to see her again, as it seems pointless giving her additional medication that she will avoid taking.

This is just an example. Keep your task simple. You could choose three or four cycles of evidence to demonstrate your competence each year.

Stage 1: Select your aspirations for good practice

The excellent GP:

- obtains informed consent to treatment
- treats patients politely and with consideration.

Stage 2: Set the standards for your outcomes

Outcomes might include:

- the way learning is applied
- a learnt skill
- a protocol
- a strategy that is implemented
- meeting recommended standards.

- A completed audit that shows that you, or all clinicians in the team, consistently obtain informed consent from patients to treatment or other clinical management.
- Devise, apply and act on an appropriate patient survey tool that ascertains patients' views about their treatment by yourself, other GPs or the practice team e.g. establishing views as to whether you treat patients politely and with consideration.
- You might choose to focus on referral to a dietitian or smoking cessation service, or the issue of concordance rather than compliance, or consent for investigations such as blood tests.

Stage 3A: Identify your learning needs

- Review the consent and communication issues in a complaint or expression of discontent made by a patient to any member of the practice team.
- Reflect on whether you follow best practice in obtaining and recording consent to treatment or procedures.

Stage 3B: Identify your service needs

> Any of the needs assessment exercises in 3A may also reveal service needs.

- Compare the consent policy in your practice against recommended best practice or another practice's consent policy and reflect on the differences.
- Audit the case notes to determine whether doctors and nurses recorded the discussion of the advantages and disadvantages of treatment and lifestyle changes in patients with hypertension.
- Undertake a targeted patient survey. You might look at patients who have consulted GPs or nurses at the surgery and had their blood pressure recorded. You could ask about any aspect of the consultation, such as whether their informed consent had been obtained before the recording, or how monitoring, treatment or lifestyle options have been explained, or their experience of consultations with the GPs or nurses, relating to politeness and consideration.

Stage 4: Make and carry out a learning and action plan

- Identify the issues from the learning and service needs assessment exercises in Stages 3A and 3B, e.g. comparing your own consent policy with others.
- Set up a workshop on communication skills highlighting politeness and consideration, and ability to gain informed consent, e.g. by video recording and reflection/feedback with various types of patients, especially those with whom you experience difficulties.
- Arrange and attend a facilitated meeting with a group of patients to discuss their experiences of consulting GPs and the practice, to gain their opinions about how well consent is explained and obtained by the clinical and non-clinical staff in the surgery e.g. organised by the practice's patient participation group.

Stage 5: Document your learning, competence, performance and standards of service delivery

- Make notes of the review of a complaint or adverse comments and subsequent plan to minimise likelihood of re-occurrence.
- Repeat the initial learning or service needs assessments, e.g. re-audit and repeat the patient survey.
- Audit that the consent policy is applied consistently by all clinical members of the practice team, e.g. from case notes, patient feedback, self-report. You

might find that consent and concordance are reported as being obtained but not recorded in the patients' records. This would imply that a change in recording practice is required and produce future new learning needs!

Box 3.2:   Case study continued

You help Mrs Humble to understand the risk and consequences of her present state of health and her present behaviour patterns. You talk through the advantages and disadvantages of medication and its long-term nature. You suggest an assertiveness course she might like to consider, run by the local further education college. You refer her to the local smoking cessation service for support and help with stopping smoking as the first step in gaining control over her adverse lifestyle.

Example cycle of evidence 3.2

- Focus: informed consent
- Other relevant foci: research; relationships with patients

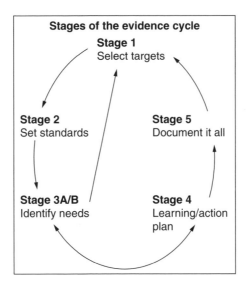

Stages of the evidence cycle

Stage 1
Select targets

Stage 2
Set standards

Stage 5
Document it all

Stage 3A/B
Identify needs

Stage 4
Learning/action plan

Box 3.3:   Case study

You agree as a practice to undertake a survey to find out if patients with early dementia are satisfied with your service. The practice manager will organise it, but you are nominated to lead the work. You are not sure how to survey them. You think many of the patients with early dementia are unlikely to answer questionnaires sent through the post and think you will use one of the reception staff, who has done some market research work, to interview them. You are not sure if you are getting into research territory or if it is okay to claim that you are auditing your services.

> This is just an example. Keep your task simple. You could choose three or four cycles of evidence to demonstrate your competence each year.

Stage 1: Select your aspirations for good practice

The excellent GP:

- protects patients' rights and makes sure that they are not disadvantaged by taking part in research
- gives patients the information they need about their problem in a way they can understand as a basis for informed consent.

Stage 2: Set the standards for your outcomes

Outcomes might include:

- the way learning is applied
- a learnt skill
- a protocol
- a strategy that is implemented
- meeting recommended standards.

- Informed consent policy of practice covers patients' participation in audit and research as well as consent to clinical treatment.
- You should be able to describe the difference between audit of clinical management and service provision and research.

Stage 3A: Identify your learning needs

- Read through the frequently asked questions and answers on the Department of Health website relating to research governance.[8] Consider whether you are able to answer the questions before reading the answers.
- Describe an audit plan that involves obtaining the views of standards of services by interviewing people with early dementia. Submit the plan to the chair of the local research ethics committee to check that he/she agrees that the audit proposal does not fall within the definition of research and to approve the patient literature and the process inviting informed consent to take part.

Stage 3B: Identify your service needs

Any of the needs assessment exercises in 3A may also reveal service needs.

- Draw up a leaflet to provide information about the survey for people with early dementia. Ask a research colleague for the extent to which it conforms to best practice for informed consent. Design the information leaflet so that they can give informed consent to the interview to obtain their views and audio recording of the interview.
- Ask a colleague to peer review the extent to which advice and information you give to people with early dementia during a consultation is accurate. The person involved would need to have given prior, written informed consent for the peer review (and audio recording if used).

Stage 4: Make and carry out a learning and action plan

- Obtain and read documents about research governance from the Department of Health website or from your PCO – as in section 3A (first point).[8]
- Study the application form for the ethical approval of a research study.
- Understand the limits to obtaining patients' views as part of audit of clinical and service management by reading up on informed consent. Read the GMC's booklet: *Seeking Patients' Consent: the ethical considerations.*[3] Look at whether you are explaining the details of the diagnosis or prognosis, giving an explanation of likely benefits and side-effects, explaining whether a proposed treatment is experimental and whether a doctor in training will be involved.
- Ask for a short tutorial from your local clinical governance lead about good practice in obtaining patients' views through audit, research and patient involvement activities – including good practice in informed consent.

Stage 5: Document your learning, competence, performance and standards of service delivery

- Make a comparison of your own practice with the answers to the frequently asked questions on the Department of Health website relating to research governance.[8]
- File a response letter from the chair of the local research ethics committee about the audit proposal.
- Keep the subsequent revised audit plan to ensure that work does not fall within the definition of research.
- Keep the revised patient's informed consent leaflet, following the critique.
- Repeat the peer review by the same, or another, colleague of the extent to which advice and information you give to people with early dementia during consultations is accurate.

Box 3.4:   Case study continued

The chair of the research ethics committee advises you that your plan should be classed as research rather than audit as it involves contact with patients outside their usual NHS care. He explains about the risks of using an untrained interviewer. He draws attention to the problems you might have with ensuring that those patients you are inviting to be interviewed fully understand and are able to consent to participation, and that they understand that their refusal will not prejudice their medical care. He advises you to send an application form for formal approval to the ethics committee and to contact the research lead in your PCO in line with the research governance framework if you wish to continue to develop a research project. You revise your plans as the scale of the work required is becoming out of all proportion.

Example cycle of evidence 3.3

- Focus: informed consent
- Other relevant focus: working with colleagues

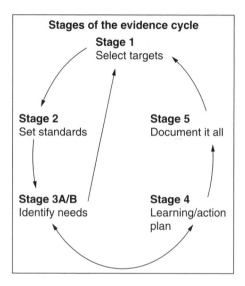

Stages of the evidence cycle

Stage 1
Select targets

Stage 2
Set standards

Stage 5
Document it all

Stage 3A/B
Identify needs

Stage 4
Learning/action
plan

Box 3.5:   Case study

Miss Younger comes with her carer to see you. The carer explains that the new manager of the unit for people with learning disabilities, in which Miss Younger lives, wants Miss Younger to have a health check-up and blood tests to establish if she is on the right dose of medication for her epilepsy. Miss Younger is 42 years old but she has not had her blood pressure or any review of her epilepsy treatment recorded. Miss Younger keeps getting up and going over to the door and does not seem to want to be there. You wonder how to proceed, as Miss Younger does not seem to have any say in this.

This is just an example. Keep your task simple. You could choose three or four cycles of evidence to demonstrate your competence each year.

Stage 1: Select your aspirations for good practice

The excellent GP:

- acts in the best interests of patients when providing or arranging treatment or care, acting with patients' informed consent
- makes sure that others understand their professional status and speciality, what roles and responsibilities they have and who is responsible for each aspect of the patient's care.

Stage 2: Set the standards for your outcomes

Outcomes might include:

- the way learning is applied
- a learnt skill
- a protocol
- a strategy that is implemented
- meeting recommended standards.

- Publish a practice policy on informed consent for patients with mental health problems and learning disabilities, including dementia.

Stage 3A: Identify your learning needs

- Analyse a significant event, e.g. you referred Miss Younger for a blood test and she refuses to co-operate resulting in telephoned protest from the phlebotomist.
- Self-assessment – you are aware that you do not know how to proceed (e.g. in the consultation in the case study). You do not know how much you can rely on the carer having already gained Miss Younger's informed consent or the extent to which you can take Miss Younger's acquiescence for 'consent'.
- Read up and reflect on the association between competency or capacity to be well informed and the degree of previous education. Also, look at the inability to provide informed consent in some individuals who have educational, social and cultural difficulties that limit their understanding of complex issues.

Stage 3B: Identify your service needs

> Any of the needs assessment exercises in 3A may also reveal service needs.

- Carry out a review of case notes of people aged 20–65 years old with learning disabilities, to determine the numbers who have had health checks, immunisations, and a recent review of the medication that they are receiving.
- Arrange a focus group discussion with people with learning disabilities and their carers to discuss the appropriateness of the patient's consent process for all clinical interventions including health checks.

Stage 4: Make and carry out a learning and action plan

- Ask for advice from MENCAP about the approach they recommend for obtaining informed consent from 'vulnerable' groups of people, how to explain clinical management and pursue clinical interventions, together with any associated useful literature.
- Read up on informed consent.
- Revise the practice informed consent policy to include specific groups of 'vulnerable' people such as those with learning disabilities or mental ill-health problems.

Stage 5: Document your learning, competence, performance and standards of service delivery

- Run a quiz for members of the practice team at an in-house educational event with four hypothetical cases. Compare the answers with best practice according to the literature available and from MENCAP.[9]
- Include the revised practice policy on informed consent.
- Audit the consistent application of the revised practice informed consent policy with consecutive cases, e.g. search on people coded as having learning disability on the computer. Look to see what interventions have been under-taken and whether informed consent has been recorded in the notes.
- Include specimen consent forms that have been piloted, revised and audited.

Box 3.6:   Case study continued

Miss Younger returns for a follow-up appointment, having left after the last surgery appointment to think about having a health check and a blood test. She has told her carer that she wants to have her health check but she does not want to have a blood test. Her most recent epileptic attack was more than 12 months ago and you agree to postpone the blood test for further discussion later. You join forces with the practice nurse to introduce her role in the health checks and take enough time to explain and start some of the checks. Miss Younger agrees to re-attend to finish the rest of the well-person screening. You arrange this so that she attends both you and the practice nurse and you can discuss her medication again.

Confidentiality

Key points

You should have appropriate confidentiality safeguards in place in the practice to prevent inadvertent disclosure of personal and sensitive information about patients. Tell people, especially the young, about their right to confidential medical treatment and reinforce your conversation with posters and leaflets. People with non-prescription drug-related problems who seek help from substance abuse clinics, or those with sexually transmitted infections who attend genitourinary medicine clinics, often do not want their GP to be told because they do not believe that the information will be kept confidential. Fears about confidentiality are the commonest reason young people give for not attending their GP for contraceptive treatment.[10]

Young people under the age of 16 years have the same rights to confidentiality as other patients. The younger the person, the greater care is needed to assess the level of understanding to ensure that he or she understands the consequences of any proposed action. If a young person fulfils the conditions given in Box 3.7 he or she is regarded as being competent to make his or her own decisions.

Occasionally you may feel that you have a moral obligation to divulge confidential information. Whenever possible you should seek to persuade the patient to give consent to the disclosure. Seek advice from your professional organisations in circumstances where others are in danger (e.g. risk of harm, or rape or sexual abuse), or where a serious crime has been committed. Health professionals should satisfy themselves that sufficient authority has been obtained (e.g. a certificate from the Attorney General or Lord Advocate) and consult professional organisations before disclosing information without a patient's consent.

Box 3.7: The Fraser Guidelines[11]

The guidelines were drawn up after Lord Fraser stated in 1985 that a doctor could give contraceptive advice or treatment to a person under 16 years old without parental consent, providing that the doctor is satisfied that:

* the young person will understand the advice
* the young person cannot be persuaded to tell their parents or allow the doctor to tell them that they are seeking contraceptive advice
* the young person is likely to begin or continue having unprotected sex with or without contraceptive treatment
* the young person's physical or mental health is likely to suffer unless they receive contraceptive advice or treatment
* it is in the young person's best interest to receive contraceptive advice or treatment.

The Fraser Guidelines apply to health professionals in England and Wales. In Scotland, the Age of Legal Capacity (Scotland) Act 1991 gives similar powers of consent to those under 16 years of age.

In Northern Ireland, although separate legislation applies, the then Department of Health and Social Services Northern Ireland stated that there was no reason to suppose that the Northern Ireland Courts would not follow the House of Lords' decision.

The Caldicott Committee Report[12] described principles of good practice to safeguard confidentiality when information is being used for non-clinical purposes:[12]

* justify the purpose
* do not use patient-identifiable information unless it is absolutely necessary
* use the minimum necessary patient-identifiable information
* access to patient-identifiable information should be on a strict need-to-know basis
* everyone with access to patient-identifiable information should be aware of his or her responsibilities.

Interpreters should be used wherever possible to avoid the use of friends or relatives. They should be trained in the requirements of confidentiality.

Patients are entitled to access data held about them. Exceptions to this right are:

* the patient failed to make the request in accordance with the Data Protection Act 1998
* if acceding to the request would result in disclosure of information about somebody else without their consent

- when giving medical information may cause serious harm to the mental or physical health of the patient (a rare occurrence).

You need to incorporate systems for ensuring that paper and computer security are maintained. Systems for monitoring and upgrading security systems should be in place and you should check regularly that confidentiality is not being breached if changes are made.

Collecting data to demonstrate your learning, competence, performance and standards of service delivery: confidentiality

Example cycle of evidence 3.4

- Focus: confidentiality
- Other relevant focus: teaching and training

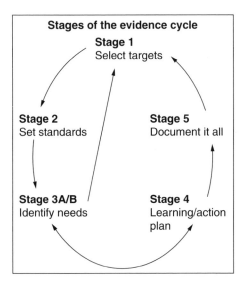

Stages of the evidence cycle

Stage 1
Select targets

Stage 2
Set standards

Stage 5
Document it all

Stage 3A/B
Identify needs

Stage 4
Learning/action plan

Box 3.9: Case study

It is the first time you have had students placed with you and you want to teach two of them about the importance of making sure that people understand the practice code on confidentiality while they are on their placement with you.

This is just an example. Keep your task simple. You could choose three or four cycles of evidence to demonstrate your competence each year.

Stage 1: Select your aspirations for good practice

The excellent GP:

- maintains the confidentiality of patient-specific information
- ensures that patients are not put at risk when seeing students or doctors in training.

Stage 2: Set the standards for your outcomes

Outcomes might include:

- the way learning is applied
- a learnt skill
- a protocol
- a strategy that is implemented
- meeting recommended standards.

- Ensure that all members of the practice team including you, new members of staff and students or doctors in training are familiar with guidelines for confidentiality in relation to patients receiving healthcare.

Stage 3A: Identify your learning needs

- Assess your knowledge about the limits of confidentiality, e.g. for providing under-16 year olds with contraception or referring them for termination of pregnancy or other surgical intervention, or for providing carers or relatives with information about a patient's condition or treatment.

- Ask an expert tutor's opinion about the particular method of teaching you plan to use for an in-house training session on maintaining confidentiality for people of different ages that will best convey main messages and lead to changes where necessary.

Stage 3B: Identify your service needs

> Any of the needs assessment exercises in 3A may also reveal service needs.

- Compare the practice protocol for confidentiality with the guidelines in the *Confidentiality and Young People* toolkit.[10]
- Review the intended induction programme for new members of staff, students on placement and doctors in training to assess the extent to which knowledge of confidentiality features and is addressed.

Stage 4: Make and carry out a learning and action plan

- Find out from the local educational tutor how to undertake learning needs assessments of others from different disciplines with different levels of responsibilities in respect of confidentiality.
- Prepare for and run an interactive teaching session on confidentiality for patients of all age groups with special focus on teenagers. You might invite the whole practice team, including students, family planning or school nurses, local pharmacists, GP registrars, etc. You could use the *Confidentiality and Young People* toolkit for promoting discussion with the practice team at the session.[10]

Stage 5: Document your learning, competence, performance and standards of service delivery

- Run a quiz completed by those attending the teaching session before and after training about confidentiality.
- Create an incident record kept by the practice team of any reported or perceived breaches of confidentiality by anyone working in, or associated with, the practice.
- Ensure the existence of personal learning plans based on learning needs assessments for new staff or doctors in training by the end of their induction period.
- Revise the practice protocol in line with the *Confidentiality and Young People* toolkit.[10]

> **Box 3.10:** Case study continued
>
> Other staff colleagues join your teaching session with the students using the video from the *Confidentiality and Young People* toolkit.[10] All get full marks in the quiz after watching the video.

Learning from complaints

Key points

There is learning to be had from every complaint. The GMC received a record 5539 complaints in 2002, 4% more than in 2001; of these, 72 resulted in a doctor being banned or suspended.[13] Even if the complaint is trivial or undeserved, it implies a lack of communication. Table 3.1 describes the nature of claims against GPs reported in a study of 1000 consecutive clinical cases. There are a myriad of associated reasons for the claims. Many of the clinical events will reveal failings in the practice systems and processes and in the practice of the GP – such as communication, diagnostic skills, etc.

Table 3.1: The nature of 1000 claims against GPs handled by the Medical Protection Society[14]

Claim by patient	Number of claims
Problems of diagnosis (delayed or missed)	631
Prescribing errors	193
Malignant neoplasms (some of the problems of diagnosis)	140
Cancer of the breast (lumpiness often falsely diagnosed as benign)	20
Cancer of the cervix (often abnormalities are filed away and not acted upon)	14
Cancer of the digestive organs (cancer of the colon most frequent with misdiagnosed symptoms)	21
Diabetes (8 deaths) primary failure to diagnose (19 delays in diagnosis; 9 delays in referral of patient resulting in amputation)	40
Myocardial infarction 27 deaths (8 undiagnosed, 7 diagnosed as dyspepsia, 3 diagnosed as congestive cardiac failure, 3 as muscular origin, 2 as chest infection)	34
Prescribing	
Steroids (e.g. osteoporotic collapse)	40
Antibiotic allergy	8
Phenothiazines (extrapyramidal symptoms)	10
Hormone replacement therapy	9
Oral contraception	9
Warfarin (interactions e.g. resulting in cerebral haemorrhage)	5

Collecting data to demonstrate your learning, competence, performance and standards of service delivery: complaints

Example cycle of evidence 3.5

- Focus: complaints
- Other relevant focus: working with colleagues

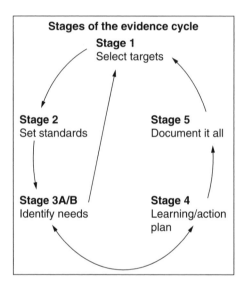

Stages of the evidence cycle

Stage 1
Select targets

Stage 2
Set standards

Stage 5
Document it all

Stage 3A/B
Identify needs

Stage 4
Learning/action plan

Box 3.11:   Case study

Your practice has received a patient complaint about a GP locum failing to diagnose a patient's shingles on the first occasion they consulted, resulting in persistent post-herpetic pain. This has prompted you all as a practice team to review the way that your complaints system functions.

This is just an example. Keep your task simple. You could choose three or four cycles of evidence to demonstrate your competence each year.

Stage 1: Select your aspirations for good practice

The excellent GP:

- apologises appropriately when things go wrong, and has an adequate complaints procedure in place.

Stage 2: Set the standards for your outcomes

Outcomes might include:

- the way learning is applied
- a learnt skill
- a protocol
- a strategy that is implemented
- meeting recommended standards.

- Understand and establish effective processes for preventing and managing complaints from patients in the practice.

Stage 3A: Identify your learning needs

- Examine as a significant event one or more complaints, e.g. where the practice has not advised a patient correctly about the complaints process.
- Compare the actual care of a patient against an acceptable standard of care for a range of clinical conditions as ongoing review for a clinical area that has been the subject of a complaint (e.g. treatment of herpes zoster as in the case study). You could use peer review by asking respected colleagues or compare your practice against a published standard such as a guideline by a responsible body of professional opinion.

Stage 3B: Identify your service needs

Any of the needs assessment exercises in 3A may also reveal service needs.

- Audit patient complaints in the preceding 12 months: the number, the outcomes and how the complaint system is advertised, etc.
- Audit the extent to which doctors and nurses are following practice agreed protocols. This is about being proactive about preventing or minimising the likelihood of the source of the complaint recurring.

- Audit vulnerable areas. Look back at the analysis of complaints to identify useful areas for focusing learning, e.g. a review of the prescribing of steroids.
- Review the way that the qualifications of locums are checked and that they are made aware of the practice protocols.

Stage 4: Make and carry out a learning and action plan

- Ask your PCO to look at the practice complaints system and feed back how it can be improved (if at all).
- Arrange a tutorial between the practice manager and others in the team about preventing and managing complaints, or use one of the risk management packages produced by medical defence organisations.[15,16]
- Read up on how to undertake significant event analysis including how to share the information with the practice team and respond as a practice team.

Stage 5: Document your learning, competence, performance and standards of service delivery

- Collect evidence of clinical competence to guard against a complaint.
- Develop a protocol of the patient complaint process against which consecutive complaints can be audited in another 12 months' time.
- Document guidance about physical examinations including that the reason for any examination should be communicated clearly, that a chaperone should be offered for any genital or breast examination, and the comfort and privacy of the patient should always be kept in mind to avoid potential complaints.
- Make sure a file containing practice protocols is available for easy reference on the desktop of the computer.

Box 3.12:   Case study continued

You are invited by your PCO to take a lead in advising GPs in other practices about the handling of complaints. They were impressed by the way your complaint system was applied when you invited them to visit your practice and advise about the handling of complaints.

References

1 Chambers R and Wakley G (2000) *Making Clinical Governance Work for You.* Radcliffe Medical Press, Oxford.

2 British Medical Association and Association of British Insurers (2002) *Medical Information and Insurance.* British Medical Association, London. See www.bma.org.uk/ap.nsf/Content/MedicalInfoInsurance.

3 General Medical Council (2002) *Seeking Patients' Consent: the ethical considerations.* General Medical Council, London.

4 Elwyn G, Edwards A and Britten N (2003) 'Doing prescribing': how doctors can be more effective. *British Medical Journal.* **327**: 864–7.

5 Heath I (2003) A wolf in sheep's clothing: a critical look at the ethics of drug taking. *British Medical Journal.* **327**: 856–8.

6 Townsend A, Hunt K and Wyke S (2003) Managing multiple morbidity in mid-life: a qualitative study of attitudes to drug use. *British Medical Journal.* **327**: 837–40.

7 Sanz EJ (2003) Concordance and children's use of medicines. *British Medical Journal.* **327**: 858–60.

8 http://www.dh.gov.uk/PolicyAndGuidance/ResearchAndDevelopment/fs/en.

9 www.mencap.org.uk.

10 Royal College of General Practitioners and Brook (2000) *Confidentiality and Young People. A toolkit for general practice, primary care groups and trusts.* Royal College of General Practitioners, London.

11 The Fraser Guidelines (1985) House of Lords Judgement, London.

12 Department of Health (1997) Report of the review of patient-identifiable information. In: *The Caldicott Committee Report.* Department of Health, London.

13 General Medical Council (2003) *Fitness to Practise Statistics for 2002.* General Medical Council, London.

14 Panting G (2003) *Nature of 1000 Claims against GPs.* Medical Protection Society, London (presentation at primary care conference, Birmingham).

15 MPS Risk Consulting, Granary Wharf House, Leeds LS11 5PY or http://www.mps-riskconsulting.com.

16 MDU Services Ltd, 230 Blackfriars Road, London SE1 8PJ or http://www.the-mdu.com.

4

Cardiovascular disease

Box 4.1: Case study

Mr Export attends asking for advice about how to reduce his risks of heart disease. His father has just had a stent put in for a narrowed coronary artery. Mr Export used to be very active, but since he took a promotion at work has not found the time for regular exercise. He is now aged 42 years and has not attended the surgery since he broke his leg when in his thirties. He looks like a rugby player gone to seed and you confirm he is obese at a BMI of 35. His blood pressure (160/92 mmHg with a large cuff) is not optimal either. He tells you that he has never smoked and his alcohol consumption has decreased to very small amounts since his promotion – the American company he works for disapproves of excess alcohol. You discuss with him how to increase his exercise levels again and reduce his weight. You arrange for fasting glucose and a lipid profile, as his father told him that he is on medication for cholesterol. You make him another appointment to discuss his results and check his blood pressure again.

What issues you should cover

Reducing Mr Export's risk of coronary artery disease will also reduce his risks of arteriosclerotic disease elsewhere in the body, including peripheral vascular disease and ischaemic stroke. Cardiovascular disease is a major cause of premature death in most European and North American populations. The underlying cause of death is thought to be arteriosclerosis, which develops gradually over many years without symptoms until the condition is advanced. Myocardial infarction, stroke and death may occur suddenly in situations remote from medical care. Modification of risk factors has been shown to reduce mortality and morbidity.[1]

Clinical priorities

The current strategy for medical intervention is to focus on those who are at highest risk of coronary heart disease:

- primary prevention for individuals at high absolute risk of developing arteriosclerosis
- secondary prevention for those with established cardiovascular disease.

More general population approaches such as reducing smoking by legislative action, promoting healthy eating, increasing exercise and reducing obesity are likely to have greater effects on long-term risk levels in the whole population. Health professionals can influence these initiatives made by governmental and non-governmental bodies, but cannot be wholly responsible for their implementation.

Assessment of risk

Absolute risk is the probability of developing coronary heart disease over a defined period. It can be established using risk prediction charts, of which there are a bewildering number.[2–5] These include:

- The Sheffield Table[4]
- New Zealand Guidelines[5]
- The Joint British Chart[2,3]
- Systematic Coronary Risk Evaluation (SCORE) – the most recent one produced by the European Cardiac Society.[1]

Most clinical computer systems have a chart available for use, or one can be downloaded from the web.

Risk factors for coronary heart disease are

- hypertension
- smoking
- high levels of total and low density lipoproteins (LDL)
- low levels of high density lipoproteins (HDL)
- diabetes
- increasing age in males of all ages and postmenopausal females
- family history of cardiovascular disease at an early age.

Established coronary heart disease, stroke or peripheral vascular disease make someone a high risk automatically and a candidate for secondary preventive measures.

Risk factors may be multifactorial, or someone may have a very high level of one risk factor. An individual with diabetes or familial hypercholesteraemia would have a high risk even without any other risk factors.

Magnetic resonance imaging (MRI) can identify atheromatous plaques in arteries and computed tomography (CT) can quantify the size of calcified deposits. Ultrasound of the carotid artery wall can also be used to detect thickening and an increased risk. These methods may become more precise in the future for the determination of risk.

Behavioural change

It is difficult, but not impossible, to help people make significant changes in their health behaviour. It is harder for people to change if they are socially disadvantaged or poor, are unemployed or in jobs without any control of their situation, and under stress at work or home. Targeting the lifestyle changes to prevent cardiovascular disease requires that someone is interested in changing, progresses to preparation to change, and then to making changes. People may relapse after making changes and need encouragement to repeat the process and maintain the changes made.[6]

Smoking

There is no safe level of smoking. All patients should be advised to stop and you can refer them to a local smoking cessation service if available.

Healthy eating

A good diet can modify several risk factors. It can reduce excess weight and blood pressure, control glucose levels, alter the ratio between high and low density lipoproteins, reduce triglyceride levels and reduce the likelihood of thrombosis. General recommendations include advice to:

- control the total intake to match the energy expenditure, once excess weight has been lost
- increase the proportion of foods in the categories that are helpful: fruit and vegetables, whole grain cereals and bread, low fat dairy produce like skimmed milk, fish and lean meat
- include oily fish and omega-3 fatty acids (that have been shown to reduce mortality after a heart attack)
- keep the total fat intake to no more than a third of the total intake. Make at least two-thirds of the fat intake unsaturated fats. Replace saturated fats partly with complex carbohydrates, and partly with monounsaturated and polyunsaturated fats from vegetable and fish sources
- reduce salt intake
- reduce excess alcohol, but one to two units of alcohol daily have a protective effect.

Physical activity

Advise all patients without contraindications to take at least 20–30 minutes of vigorous exercise most days of the week. More moderate exercise is still of benefit, if this cannot be achieved because of other health problems. Moderate to high activity significantly reduces coronary heart disease and stroke.[4]

Medication

Assess Mr Export's total cardiovascular risk. Treatment should be aimed at those with more than a 3% per annum risk of an event or more than a 30% ten-year absolute risk. Various guides are available for this (*see* above), but the National Service Framework advises that we use the Joint British Heart Society Charts.[3,7] Medication is mainly used for those needing secondary prevention. Anybody with diabetes will be regarded as high risk.

Mr Export may want to discuss taking aspirin. The role of aspirin for primary prevention is based largely on two trials, the US Physicians' Study[8] which studied older men aged 40–84 years at relatively low risk, and the UK Thrombosis Prevention Trial which studied higher risk men aged 45–69 years.[9] Aspirin significantly reduced coronary events by 44% in the US trial and 20% in the UK trial. The five-year number needed to treat (NNT) to avert one non-fatal myocardial infarction was 105 in the US study and 83 in the UK study. Unlike secondary prevention, there was no reduction in overall cardiovascular mortality in either of these primary prevention trials. *Clinical Evidence* states that insufficient evidence was found to identify which individuals would benefit from taking aspirin.[10] Of course, some people will suffer the adverse effect of bleeding while taking aspirin or be unable to tolerate it.

Mr Export is likely to want to discuss his cholesterol levels and whether he should be taking any medication for this. Use the ratio of total cholesterol to HDL to interpret the risk charts. Many risk factor assessment tools do not take into account family history. For example, if Mr Export's father had been in his forties when he suffered a myocardial infarction this would be a significant family history and would move Mr Export from the yellow zone to the red zone (i.e. from a 15–30% risk category to more than 30% risk).

Box 4.2:   Case study continued

When Mr Export returns, he tells you that he has joined a gym across the road from his head office. He has arranged to go there every lunchtime and has entered a fitness programme. He has already started making changes to his diet, as he was sitting having sandwiches, crisps and several chocolate biscuits every lunchtime before. He has discussed his new regime with his wife, who is

continued opposite

---

keen for him to buy a bike so that they can go off at the weekend together as a family. His blood pressure is much the same and you arrange for him to attend for monitoring of his weight and blood pressure. His total cholesterol to HDL cholesterol level is 5, and you show him his risk from the Joint British Societies Risk Prediction chart. You emphasise that this is a lifelong project and that his risks will need reassessing at intervals, to ensure that he keeps his risk factors low.

Secondary prevention

Box 4.3:   Case study

Mrs Holiday asks, 'Do I need to take all of these tablets? Will I be able to stop them when I've finished this supply – the hospital said something about getting more from you? Is that right?' The discharge note from the hospital says 'troponin-positive acute coronary syndrome' followed by a long list of drugs. She tells you that she was surprised to be told she had had a heart attack. While away on a weekend break she had been woken early one morning with what she thought was bad indigestion. She rang NHS Direct for advice and after going through her symptoms, an ambulance arrived to take her to hospital. She had an ECG (electrocardiogram) and some blood tests, but had no more pain after the injections she had that day. She was discharged from hospital after four days and is to have an exercise test arranged locally. She says she feels bewildered and unsure about the future. She is 66 years old but is still working – she needs a sick note – and has never had any medical treatment except when she had her children and for occasional urinary tract infections. She never takes exercise preferring to zip around in her little car, she only smokes 'socially' but drinks and eats well.

Lifestyle advice

You would start by going through with Mrs Holiday what she can do to control her risk factors in much the same way as for Mr Export (above). This will help her to feel that she is more in control of her illness. If she needs nicotine replacement therapy to help her stop smoking, this seems to be safe in people with coronary artery disease.[10]

Give her a leaflet to back up your advice – the patient information leaflets (PILs) from Prodigy are clear and succinct without any promotional material.[11] Tell her that she is likely to feel tired and have some aches and pains for a week or so. She should begin physical activity gently, but gradually increase over

4–6 weeks. Most people get back to work within 2–3 months but she will need to be guided by how she feels and the type of work she does – she will need to take longer if her work is physically demanding. If she is able to walk without discomfort, then a return to sexual activity should not cause any problems. She can resume car driving after 4–6 weeks provided she has made a satisfactory recovery (and her insurance company is happy). Air travel (as a passenger, that is) should also be alright. Public service vehicle and heavy goods vehicle licensing rules are stricter and further assessment would be required.

Cardiac rehabilitation

Cardiac rehabilitation can reduce the risk of death and further myocardial infarction. The programme provides advice and help on exercise, diet, stress, and other aspects of getting back into full health following a heart attack. It is also useful to mix with others who are going through the same experience.[6]

Drug treatment[10]

Go through with her what she has been prescribed and explain the reasons for each preparation. It is important that she understands why she needs to take the drugs so that she feels sure that this is what she wants to do (*see* concordance, Chapter 3).

Antiplatelet medication

Low dose aspirin (75 mg per day) reduces the risk of another episode of myocardial infarction, stroke or other vascular thrombosis. The benefits outweigh the risk of both cerebral and gastrointestinal haemorrhage. Other antiplatelet drugs, e.g. clopidogrel, are very much more expensive and are usually only used if aspirin is contraindicated. Indigestion is the commonest side-effect and, in patients at high risk, aspirin can be combined with a proton pump inhibitor. This combination may be more successful than other antiplatelet medications as they also tend to cause indigestion.

Beta-blocking drugs

Treatment with beta-blocking drugs reduces total mortality, sudden death and reduces the risk of another myocardial infarction. There is no clear evidence that any one type of beta-blocker is any better than another, so look for the lowest price that suits that patient. Remember that asthma is a contraindication to beta-blockers and about a quarter of people started on them suffer ill effects.[10]

Lipid-lowering drugs

Statins are the single most effective type of treatment for reducing cholesterol levels and reducing cardiovascular risk. Immediately after a myocardial infarction, a temporary reduction in cholesterol levels occurs, so measurement about 6–12 weeks after the event gives a better guide. Most patients who have a myocardial infarction will be started on a statin. Contraindications include liver disease and porphyria, so liver function must be monitored. Statins interact with other drugs broken down in the liver, macrolide antibiotics such as erythromycin, and with grapefruit juice.

The Heart Protection Study was a UK-based study in over 20 000 patients reported in 2002.[12] It looked at patients aged 40–80 years of age who had not only existing coronary heart disease, but also peripheral vascular disease, stroke or diabetes. Adding simvastatin to existing treatments produced substantial additional benefits for a wide range of high-risk patients, irrespective of their initial cholesterol concentrations. Allocation to 40 mg simvastatin daily reduced the rates of myocardial infarction, and of stroke, by about one-quarter. After making allowance for non-compliance, actual use of this regimen would probably reduce these rates by about one-third. The study showed that among the many types of high-risk individual studied, simvastatin would prevent about 70–100 people per 1000, over the 5 years of treatment, from suffering at least one of these major vascular events, and longer treatment should produce further benefit. The size of the 5-year benefit depends chiefly on such individuals' overall risk of major vascular events, rather than on their blood lipid concentrations alone. The benefit seen was in addition to the benefit of aspirin, beta-blockers and angiotensin converting enzyme (ACE) inhibitors. This study, which was the largest statin study ever conducted, has massive implications for practice and challenges the previous concept of only treating with statins if the lipids are above a certain level. The study reinforces the practice of targeting patients on their absolute risk of suffering a cardiovascular event and that statins should be an option for all those at risk, not just those with high cholesterols. This has considerable implications for the cost of these therapies for the health service.

Cost-effectiveness depends on what dose of which statin is used for each patient's particular risk profile.

Angiotensin converting enzyme inhibitors

ACE inhibitors improve left ventricular function in patients who have had a myocardial infarction. Even without evidence of left ventricular dysfunction, outcomes in terms of fewer deaths, strokes and myocardial infarctions occur in patients given ACE inhibitors.

Other medication

In selected high-risk patients, anticoagulant therapy rather than aspirin may prevent further thrombotic episodes but is associated with a significant risk of haemorrhage.[10] Amiodarone may be required for control of tachyarrhythmias and reduces the risk of sudden death in this high-risk group of patients.[10]

Patients with angina will need nitrates. For occasional glyceryl trinitrate, tablets (that need renewing every eight weeks once opened) or a spray are most convenient. Consider longer acting preparations such as isosorbide mononitrate for more regular prophylaxis.

Quality indicators in coronary heart disease

The Quality and Outcomes Framework represents a different approach to the contracting arrangements for GPs, with incentives for those that demonstrate quality improvements in key areas, both clinical and non-clinical (*see* page vii). The quality points available are achievable on a sliding scale, so as you are collecting the data to demonstrate your own competence you are also helping to show that your practice is achieving high standards of care. Some of the quality indicators will obviously overlap with those for hypertension. They include:

- a register of patients with coronary heart disease: 6 points
- 90% of patients with new onset angina referred for exercise testing or specialist assessment: 7 points
- 90% of patients on the coronary heart disease register have their smoking status recorded in the last 15 months: 7 points
- 70% of patients on the coronary heart disease register who smoke have been offered smoking cessation advice in the last 15 months: 4 points
- 90% of patients on the coronary heart disease register have a blood pressure recorded in the last 15 months: 7 points
- 70% of patients on the coronary heart disease register have a blood pressure on treatment of less than that recommended by the British Hypertension Society Guidelines (150/90 mmHg) in the last 15 months: 19 points
- 90% of patients on the coronary heart disease register have their cholesterol level recorded in the last 15 months: 7 points
- 60% of patients on the coronary heart disease register have a cholesterol level on treatment of 5 mmol/l or less in the last 15 months: 16 points

- 90% of patients on the coronary heart disease register are on antithrombotic therapy in the last 15 months: 7 points
- 50% of patients on the coronary heart disease register are currently on a beta-blocker: 7 points
- 70% of patients who have had a myocardial infarction are currently on an ACE inhibitor: 7 points
- 85% of patients on the coronary heart disease register have received the influenza immunisation in the previous September to March: 7 points.

Exception reporting will be the same as for the quality targets for hypertension. That is, the patients do not wish to participate, have contraindications or unacceptable side-effects on medication, or have conditions making treatment inappropriate.

Box 4.4:   Case study continued

Mrs Holiday returns to see you after going through all the information you gave her about her future treatment. She is finding that her increased activity is causing her to have episodes of chest pain and you give advice on using nitrates. She has more questions to ask about treatment for coronary artery blockages, as she now has an appointment for an angiogram following her poor performance at exercise testing. You suggest she waits to find out the result of that first and see what options the consultant suggests. You give her the website of the British Heart Foundation as she says her granddaughter can help her to look things up.[13]

Collecting data to demonstrate your learning, competence, performance and standards of service delivery

Example cycle of evidence 4.1

- Focus: relationships with patients
- Other relevant foci: maintaining good medical practice; working with colleagues

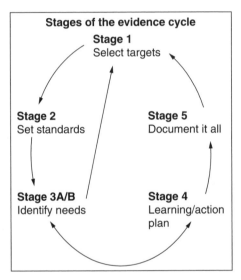

Stages of the evidence cycle

Stage 1
Select targets

Stage 2
Set standards

Stage 5
Document it all

Stage 3A/B
Identify needs

Stage 4
Learning/action plan

Box 4.5: Case study

You are surprised to see Mrs Mother, who has mild type 2 diabetes, well controlled by metformin since she lost 14 kg. One of your partners, who usually sees her, has recently reviewed her and felt she was doing very well. She takes an ACE inhibitor, a statin and aspirin. Her last recorded blood pressure at 120/72 mmHg was well within the guidelines for people with diabetes and her last blood tests for fasting glucose, her lipid profile, electrolytes and creatinine were all within normal limits. Mrs Mother attends with her son, who you have not met before. He takes over the consultation, explaining that he is over on a visit from the States where he lives. He says 'I'm just so worried about her health, nothing seems to have been done to sort it out'. He goes on to tell you that she would have had all sorts of investigations 'back home' and he can't believe that she just comes for a blood pressure check every six months and only has a blood test once a year. He wants her referred to a specialist.

This is just an example. Keep your task simple. You could choose three or four cycles of evidence to demonstrate your competence each year.

Stage 1: Select your aspirations for good practice

The excellent GP:

- empowers patients to take decisions about their management
- seeks consent before sharing information
- provides or arranges investigations or treatment when necessary
- refers to another practitioner when indicated
- keeps open lines of communication with colleagues
- works with colleagues to monitor and maintain the quality of care provided
- makes sure that others understand your professional status and speciality, what roles and responsibilities you have and who is responsible for each aspect of the patient's care.

Stage 2: Set the standards for your outcomes

Outcomes might include:

- the way learning is applied
- a learnt skill
- a protocol
- a strategy that is implemented
- meeting recommended standards.

- Demonstrate consistent best practice in the prevention of cardiovascular disease in patients who are at increased risk.
- Document best practice in managing the concerns of relatives.

Stage 3A: Identify your learning needs

- Carry out a self-assessment of your knowledge about the prevention of cardiovascular disease in patients at increased risk.
- Keep a reflective diary about how you handled your irritation over the relative's assumption that you were providing inadequate care.

- Decide how best to obtain consent to disclosure of medical information when a relative accompanies a patient.

Stage 3B: Identify your service needs

> Any of the needs assessment exercises in 3A may also reveal service needs.

- Look at the practice guidelines for review of patients at increased risk of cardiovascular disease.
- Review the practice policy for managing requests for referral to a specialist when the health professional involved is not the usual one caring for the patient.

Stage 4: Make and carry out a learning and action plan

- Compare your knowledge about the prevention of cardiovascular disease in patients at increased risk with an authoritative source you obtain and read.
- Discuss the practice guidelines for review of patients at increased risk of cardiovascular disease at a practice meeting.
- Attend a workshop on best practice on consent to disclosure of medical information and managing the concerns of relatives.
- Discuss with colleagues how to manage requests for referral from relatives, and requests to health professionals not usually responsible for the care of that patient.

Stage 5: Document your learning, competence, performance and standards of service delivery

- Record the practice guidelines (with any revisions agreed) for review of patients at increased risk of cardiovascular disease.
- Collect feedback from other health professionals about how they manage requests for referral from relatives, and from health professionals not usually responsible for the care of that patient.
- Make notes from the workshop on best practice on consent to disclosure of medical information and managing the concerns of relatives.
- Keep notes from your reflective diary.

Box 4.6:   Case study continued

You thank Mrs Mother's son for his concern. You ask Mrs Mother directly what worries *she* has about her condition and her care. She tells you that she was quite satisfied with her care until her son worried her that she might suddenly have a heart attack and told her she should have had an angiogram. You suggest that she might like some more information about how her condition is being managed and discuss it with her son at home. Then she could return to see her usual doctor, or yourself, to discuss whether she would like any alternative action to be taken. You ask if she would like a copy of her most recent tests so that she can discuss those with her son if she wishes. You arrange for the practice guidelines, the information from Prodigy,[11] and her tests results to be copied for her. You also jot down for her the names of some booklets e.g. *Understanding Coronary Heart Disease*, published in the Family Doctor Series and obtainable from most pharmacies or from www.familydoctor.co.uk. You tell your colleague about the consultation so that he is aware of the possible future request for referral and further investigations.

Example cycle of evidence 4.2

- Focus: clinical care
- Other relevant foci: working with colleagues; relationships with patients; probity

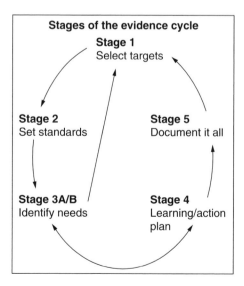

Box 4.7: Case study

Dr Count has agreed to be the lead clinician for the area of cardiovascular disease in her practice. The practice already has a disease register for coronary heart disease and for myocardial infarction that has recently been reviewed for accuracy ready for quality points. While reviewing the data for claiming points for the medication the patients on the coronary heart disease register are receiving, she is concerned to find that she cannot verify the claim that all patients are receiving aspirin, other antiplatelet medication, warfarin, or should be excluded because they have contraindications. She finds that evidence about non-smokers is easy to establish as it only needs to be recorded once. However, many of the records about current smoking are very out of date and it cannot be established whether smokers are receiving advice or have had their status checked.

This is just an example. Keep your task simple. You could choose three or four cycles of evidence to demonstrate your competence each year.

Stage 1: Select your aspirations for good practice

The excellent GP has:

- a structured approach for managing long-term health problems and preventive care.

Stage 2: Set the standards for your outcomes

Outcomes might include:

- the way learning is applied
- a learnt skill
- a protocol
- a strategy that is implemented
- meeting recommended standards.

- Every patient on the disease register for coronary heart disease has a record of antiplatelet or anticoagulant therapy or the reason for exclusion.
- Every patient who smokes and is on the disease register for coronary heart disease has a record of their smoking status and the advice given at their six monthly review.

Stage 3A: Identify your learning needs

- Self-assess your knowledge of the indications and contraindications for treatment with antiplatelets and anticoagulants in cardiovascular disease.
- Conduct a patient survey: ask ten consecutive patients who smoke (some of whom should be on the coronary heart disease register) if they have received advice about smoking within the previous two years, and if so, how appropriate the advice was perceived to be, when it had been given and by whom.

Stage 3B: Identify your service needs

Any of the needs assessment exercises in 3A may also reveal service needs.

- Audit the smoking status of patients on the coronary heart disease register for: existence of records of smoking status in the last 12 months, the extent of advice and support or help offered, and the change of smoking behaviour since the last review.
- Examine the pathway by which aspirin bought over the counter and contraindications to antiplatelet and anticoagulant medication are recorded in the electronic medical record.

Stage 4: Make and carry out a learning and action plan

- Read up about risks of smoking and provision of best practice in motivating people to stop smoking.
- Talk to smokers at an informal group, e.g. in the waiting room during influenza immunisation, and actively listen to their feedback about improving services and the quality and extent of the advice they have received about stopping smoking.
- Contact other practices with the same computer software to establish best practice in recording use of aspirin and other antiplatelet medication and the exclusion criteria for these and anticoagulant therapy.

Stage 5: Document your learning, competence, performance and standards of service delivery

- Re-audit records of patients on the coronary heart disease register to establish whether the changes in recording use or exclusion criteria concerning antiplatelet and anticoagulant therapy have been successful.
- Document a practice protocol relating to smoking cessation.
- Re-audit recording in the records of patients on the coronary heart disease register of smoking status, extent of advice and support or help offered, and the number who have changed their smoking behaviour.

- Make notes on the informal feedback from the smokers about their experiences.

Box 4.8:   Case study continued

After 12 months, the re-audit results show the results after the changes made. The data now back up the assertion that all patients on the coronary heart disease register are on antiplatelet or anticoagulant medication or have recorded exclusion criteria. Dr Count is also pleased to see that the smoking cessation efforts appear to be making small numbers of people at risk change their smoking habits. The other GPs are pleased to hear that they can substantiate their claim for quality points.

Example cycle of evidence 4.3

- Focus: teaching and training
- Other relevant foci: relationships with patients; maintaining good medical practice

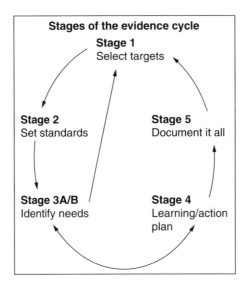

Stages of the evidence cycle

Stage 1
Select targets

Stage 2
Set standards

Stage 5
Document it all

Stage 3A/B
Identify needs

Stage 4
Learning/action plan

Box 4.9: Case study

A medical student is sitting in your surgery when Mrs Herbal arrives. Mrs Herbal is aged 43 years and has a strong family history of heart disease. She attends quite frequently complaining of headaches or feeling dizzy and asking for her blood pressure to be checked. She has had several cholesterol and blood glucose tests. All her tests have been normal. She wants to discuss taking hawthorn and garlic to prevent her developing heart disease. She would like omega-3 capsules prescribed as they are very expensive to buy. You ask the medical student if he knows about any of these medications and he says, rather abruptly, 'I'm training to be a doctor, not a herbalist'.

> This is just an example. Keep your task simple. You could choose three or four cycles of evidence to demonstrate your competence each year.

Stage 1: Select your aspirations for good practice

The excellent GP:

- helps to educate other colleagues at all levels
- does not undermine the confidence of juniors or students
- treats patients with courtesy and consideration
- keeps his/her knowledge up to date.

Stage 2: Set the standards for your outcomes

Outcomes might include:

- the way learning is applied
- a learnt skill
- a protocol
- a strategy that is implemented
- meeting recommended standards.

- Demonstrate an active involvement in the training of another.
- Behave in a courteous way to patients and students.
- Demonstrate a willingness to find out information not readily available.

Stage 3A: Identify your learning needs

- Gain peer review of your teaching skills – ask another trainer to peer review a tutorial with the medical student.
- Self-assess your awareness of the curriculum of the local medical school.
- Check that your knowledge about complementary medicines in cardio-vascular disease and prevention is up to date.
- Feedback from trainees is good way to assess your teaching, although it may be difficult to avoid bias if feedback is not anonymised.
- Check if you have the skills to guide the student to manage this type of consultation and to show him how the patient might suffer if he is perceived to be unhelpful.

Stage 3B: Identify your service needs

Any of the needs assessment exercises in 3A may also reveal service needs.

- Undertake a force-field analysis with others in the practice team about the driving and restraining factors involved in teaching medical students.

Stage 4: Make and carry out a learning and action plan

- Attend a meeting of the medical school curriculum group.
- Attend an update meeting about complementary medicines in cardio-vascular disease and prevention and read widely about the subject.
- Attend a 'Training the trainers' course or, if it is a while since you last went on a course, a refresher course may be a good idea.
- Reflect on the outcome of the force-field analysis with other teachers in the practice. Make a plan to boost the driving factors.

Stage 5: Document your learning, competence, performance and standards of service delivery

- Keep a record of your discussion with, and the feedback from, the medical student.
- Keep a record of the teaching concerning the curriculum.
- Record the outcome of the force-field analysis.
- Record your notes about your new knowledge on complementary medicines in cardiovascular disease and prevention.
- Keep a record of your notes on the trainers' course.

Box 4.10:   Case study continued

Mrs Herbal is mollified by your offer to look up the effects of hawthorn and garlic. You consult the *British National Formulary* and inform her that the omega-3 capsules are only licensed for secondary prevention after a myocardial infarction or for people with hypertriglyceraemia.[3] You add that eating oily fish three times a week would give her good protection without needing to add any expensive supplements.

   After Mrs Herbal has left, you discuss with the medical student his feeling that he does not need to know about complementary medicines. You help him to understand that patients may avoid telling a doctor about their use and put themselves at risk of side-effects or interactions, if they think the doctor will disapprove. You find the relevant summary in *Bandolier* to give to the medical student[14] and show him how you access a paper on alternative therapies and heart failure in the *American Family Physician*.[15]

References

1   Third Joint Task Force of European and other Societies on Cardiovascular Disease Prevention in Clinical Practice (2003) European Guidelines on cardiovascular disease prevention in clinical practice. *European Heart Journal.* **24**: 1601–10, www.escardio.org/scinfo/Tforceguidelines.htm.

2   Foord-Kelcey G (ed.) (2003) *Guidelines* vol. 20. Medendium Group Publishing Ltd, Berkhamsted. www.eguidelines.co.uk.

3   Joint Formulary Committee (2003) *British National Formulary*. British Medical Association and Royal Pharmaceutical Society, London. www.bnf.org.

4   Wallis EJ, Ramsay LE, Haq IU *et al.* (2000) Coronary and cardiovascular risk estimation for primary prevention: validation of a new Sheffield table in the 1995 Scottish health survey population. *British Medical Journal.* **320**: 671–6.

5   The National Heart Foundation of New Zealand, Cardiac Society of Australia and New Zealand and the Royal New Zealand College of General Practitioners Working Party (1997) New Zealand guidelines for the management of chronic heart failure. *New Zealand Medical Journal.* **110**: 99–107, www.nzgg.org.nz.

6   Chambers R, Wakley G and Iqbal Z (2001) *Cardiovascular Matters in Primary Care.* Radcliffe Medical Press, Oxford.

7   www.dh.gov.uk/assetRoot/04/04/90/70/04049070.pdf.

8   Steering Committee of the Physicians' Health Study (1989) Final report of the aspirin component of the ongoing Physicians' Health Study. *New England Journal of Medicine.* **321**: 129–35.

9   Meade TW, Brennan PJ, on behalf of the MRC General Practice Research Framework (2000) Determination of who will derive the most benefit from

aspirin in primary prevention; subgroup results from a randomised controlled trial. *British Medical Journal.* **321**: 13–17.

10   Godlee F (ed.) (2003) *Clinical Evidence.* BMJ Publishing Group, London, www.clinicalevidence.com.

11   www.prodigy.nhs.uk.

12   Heart Protection Study Collaborative Group (2002) MRC/BHF Heart Protection Study of cholesterol lowering with simvastin in 20 536 high-risk individuals: a randomised placebo-controlled trial. *Lancet.* **360**: 7–22.

13   www.bhf.org.uk.

14   www.jr2.ox.ac.uk/bandolier/booth/hliving/FishCHD2.html.

15   http://www.aafp.org/afp/20000915/1325.html.

5

Hypertension

Box 5.1: Case study

Mr Round is 48 years old. He had moved house and registered with the practice three months ago. When he had a new patient medical with the practice nurse, she had recorded his blood pressure as 170/110 mmHg. He had obediently returned twice since but his readings remained elevated at 166/104 and 168/100 mmHg. You now have his medical record from his previous general practice. He appears to have consulted very little and his only blood pressure record is nine years ago when it was 140/80 mmHg.

What issues you should cover

The case for treatment

Definitions for 'hypertension' vary according to the country and population and have changed over time.[1] The British Hypertension Guidelines[2] and the National Service Framework for Coronary Heart Disease[3] define hypertension as:

> a sustained systolic blood pressure of 140 mmHg (mercury) or more, or
> a diastolic blood pressure of 85 mmHg or more.

Systolic and diastolic pressures are continuously related to the risk of developing cardiovascular disease and the risk extends into that usually regarded as 'normal' blood pressures. A practice that can show it has measured blood pressure in adult patients within the last five years will gain quality points under the new contract. Measurements in at least 55% of patients of 45 years and over will gain ten organisational points and at least 75% coverage will gain 15 points.

In controlled trials over 3–5 years, drug treatment for hypertension prevents cardiovascular complications, but little is known about long-term prognosis. A follow-up study over 20–22 years showed that treated males with hypertension had significantly increased mortality, especially from coronary heart disease, compared with males without hypertension from the same population.[4] The high incidence of coronary heart disease was related to organ damage, smoking and cholesterol levels at the time of entry to the study. Untreated males with hypertension have an even greater risk of death or disability. The moral is do not look at levels of blood pressure in isolation – look at the whole person and their risk factors. Reducing blood pressure helps to prevent stroke, but other risk factors (e.g. smoking, cholesterol levels) are likely to be more important in preventing the other cardiovascular adverse events.

The British Hypertension Guidelines [2] and the National Service Framework for Coronary Heart Disease[3] recommend treatment for people who have:

sustained systolic blood pressure of 160 mmHg or more and/or diastolic pressure of 100 mmHg or more

and treatment at lower limits for those who have other risk factors:

sustained systolic pressure 140–159 mmHg or diastolic pressures of 85–99 mmHg.

Other risk factors include:

- evidence of established cardiovascular disease
- diabetes
- a ten-year risk of cardiovascular disease of more than 15% using one of the coronary heart risk charts (*see* Chapter 4)
- the presence of target organ damage.

Initial assessment of the patient with hypertension

Guidelines for the assessment and treatment of patients with hypertension should be up to date and accessible to all clinical staff. The British Hypertension Society guidelines appear in *Guidelines* or on the eguidelines website.[5,6]

The guidelines include that you should measure the blood pressure of all adults at least every five years until the age of 80 years. If you identify someone with a borderline value (135–139/85–89 mmHg), or if someone has had previous raised levels, check the blood pressure every year. Arrange at least two measurements at each of four visits before labelling someone as hypertensive. If Mr Round has similar elevated readings on this fourth occasion, you might justifiably label him as suffering from sustained hypertension and consider whether he requires treatment.

You should establish if Mr Round has:

- an underlying cause for hypertension (*see* Table 5.1)
- other risk factors present (smoking, obesity, diabetes, etc.)
- any complications already present (e.g. previous stroke)

- any end organ damage (e.g. left ventricular hypertrophy)
- any other conditions that might affect treatment (e.g. asthma preventing the use of beta-blockers).

Table 5.1: Underlying causes (present in about 5–10% of people with hypertension)[7]

Cause	What to look for
Drug induced	Non-steroidal anti-inflammatory drugs, corticosteroids, combined oral contraceptives, cyclosporin, erythropoietin
Endocrine	
Primary aldosteronism	Tetany, muscle weakness, polyuria, hypokalaemia
Cushing's syndrome	Truncal obesity, striae, etc.
Phaeochromocytoma	Intermittent high blood pressure, sweating attacks, palpitations
Acromegaly	Enlargement of hands and feet, coarsening of facial features, visual field loss, etc.
Vascular	
Coarctation of aorta	Delayed or weak femoral pulses
Renal artery stenosis	Peripheral vascular disease, abdominal bruit
Renal	
Chronic pyelonephritis	History of recurrent infections
Diabetic nephropathy	Microalbuminuria or proteinuria
Glomerulonephritis	Microscopic haematuria
Obstructive uropathy	Abdominal or flank mass
Polycystic kidneys	Abdominal or flank mass, microscopic haematuria, family history
Connective tissue disorders	
Scleroderma	Skin changes
Systemic lupus erythematosis	Joint pain
Polyarteritis nodosa	Fatigue and weakness
Retroperitoneal fibrosis	Abdominal pain
	Other symptoms or signs

The history and examination will point you towards most of these conditions. Investigations that might help are:

- urine strip test for blood and protein
- blood electrolytes and creatinine
- blood glucose
- ratio of serum total cholesterol to HDL cholesterol
- ECG.

The European Society of Hypertension guidelines also recommend echocardiography as a routine investigation to detect ischaemia, conduction defects and arrhythmias.[7] However, this may not be practicable in your area.

You will need to refer some patients to secondary care when they have:

- an underlying cause as they may require specialist investigations to which you do not have access
- very high blood pressure levels (more than 220/120 mmHg), accelerated rises (malignant hypertension) or impending complications
- treatment difficulties e.g. poor control on three medications, side-effects or contraindications to medication
- special problems e.g. unusually variable levels, pregnancy.

Management of established hypertension

Encourage Mr Round to make lifestyle changes (*see* Table 5.2). This may be all that is necessary in patients who have mild hypertension but no target organ damage or cardiovascular complications. Reassess after four to six months and monitor levels at yearly intervals – lifestyle changes are difficult to sustain. When drug treatment is indicated, introduce these interventions at the same time as medication. Evidence about changing behaviour shows that it *is* worth making the effort to advise people about lifestyle changes.[8] Lifestyle changes can make a substantial impact on risk factors and even small changes in weight can lower blood pressure – blood pressure readings fall by about 2.5 (systolic)/1.5 mmHg (diastolic) for each kilogram of weight loss.

Table 5.2: Non-drug treatments[8]

To lower blood pressure	To reduce the risk of cardiovascular disease
Weight reduction	Stop smoking
Take dynamic exercise like brisk walking (rather than isometric exercise like weight training)	Reduce saturated fat in the diet and replace it with polyunsaturated or monounsaturated fat
Limit alcohol to less than 3–4 units (men) or 2–3 units (women) per day	Increase the intake of oily fish
Reduce added salt or avoid salty foods	
Increase the intake of fruit and vegetables and decrease the saturated and total fat intake	

The Hypertension Optimal Treatment trial (HOT) suggested that the optimal blood pressure for reduction of cardiovascular events was 139/83 mmHg.[9] The numbers in this trial were not large and the group whose blood pressure was below 150/90 mmHg had no obvious disadvantages. Patients with diabetes had greater lowering of their risk if their diastolic blood pressure was kept below 80 mmHg. Discuss the optimal treatment with each patient as not everyone will be willing or able to achieve these targets. Record your discussion to back up any claim for exemption from your targets.

Antihypertensive drug therapy

Three long-term, double blind studies compared the major classes of antihypertensive drugs and found no consistent or important differences in efficacy, side-effects or quality of life.[2] There were differences between the classes of drugs related to ethnic group and age. Treatment trials with beta-blockers or thiazides provide most of the evidence about benefits of blood pressure lowering for reduction of cardiovascular risk. Trials of medication for hypertension have some limitations. Most patients in the trials had high additional risk factors such as diabetes, and compliance with treatment in trials is much higher than in everyday clinical practice. These controlled randomised trials lasted for 4–5 years, whereas life expectancy in middle-aged people with hypertension is 20–30 years.[7]

Consider individual patient variations when deciding on which treatment to choose (*see* Table 5.3).

Table 5.3: Major classes of drugs for treatment of patients with hypertension[2,7]

	Other conditions from which the patient is suffering			
Class of drug	*Drug of choice*	*Possible choice*	*Caution*	*Contraindicated*
Thiazide	Elderly	Good initial choice for most	Abnormal lipids	Gout
Beta-blockers	Myocardial infarction Angina	Heart failure[a]	Heart failure Abnormal lipids Peripheral vascular disease	Asthma Chronic obstructive pulmonary disease Heart block
ACE inhibitors	Heart failure Left ventricular dysfunction Type 1 diabetic nephropathy	Chronic renal disease[a] Type 2 diabetic nephropathy	Peripheral vascular disease (exclude renovascular disease)	Pregnancy Renovascular disease

continued overleaf

Table 5.3:   *continued*

| Class of drug | Other conditions from which the patient is suffering | | | |
	Drug of choice	Possible choice	Caution	Contraindicated
Angiotensin II receptor antagonists	As for ACE inhibitors but preferable if cough develops with ACE inhibitor treatment	Intolerance to other antihypertensive drugs	As for ACE inhibitors	As for ACE inhibitors
Alpha-blockers	Prostatism	Abnormal lipids	Postural hypotension	Urinary incontinence
Calcium antagonists (dihydropyridine; class II)	Isolated systolic hypertension in the elderly	Angina Elderly Afro-Caribbean	Headache Flushing Oedema	
Calcium antagonists (rate limiting; classes I and III)	Angina	Myocardial infarction	Combination with beta-blocker	Heart block Heart failure

[a]But condition may worsen, seek specialist advice

Tailor the drug regime to suit the patient whenever possible. If there are no indications to direct the first choice to specific drugs, then a low dose of a thiazide, e.g. bendrofluazide (bendroflumethiazide) 2.5 mg or hydrochlorthiazide 25 mg, is cost-effective. The dose–response curve for thiazides shows that increasing the dose does not increase efficacy, so change the type of medication, or add in another, if there is a poor response. Unless very urgent, change therapy only after an interval of about four weeks. Always check first that the patient is taking the medication. Concordance, not compliance (*see* Chapter 3), is important in treating a condition in which patients may feel less well on treatment than without.

It appears reasonable to start treatment either with a low dose of a single agent or with a low dose combination of two agents.[7] If you choose low dose single agent therapy and blood pressure control is not achieved, the next step is to switch to a low dose of a different agent. Alternatively, you could increase the dose of the first preparation chosen (with a greater possibility of causing adverse effects) or move to combination therapy. If you started with a low dose combination, you can use a higher dose combination or add a low dose of a third medication.

Many patients will need more than one type of therapy to achieve reduction of blood pressure to target levels. Try to give as few drugs as possible and preferably in a single daily dose. Multiple dosing increases the risk of forgotten tablets. Suitable combinations might be:

*   a thiazide with an ACE inhibitor
*   a beta-blocker with a calcium antagonist (dihydropyridine type)
*   a calcium antagonist with an ACE inhibitor.

Evidence is accumulating that an unacceptably high risk of a patient developing diabetes may result from combining a thiazide with a beta blocker. Guidelines under development in 2004 will no longer recommend this combination. You would obviously avoid a combination of a beta-blocker and a rate-limiting calcium channel antagonist to avoid slowing the heart rate to dangerous levels! Other combinations to avoid are an ACE inhibitor and an angiotensin II antagonist, or an ACE inhibitor with a potassium-sparing diuretic.

A commonly used third-line combination is a diuretic with an ACE inhibitor and a calcium antagonist.

Fixed dose combinations may be sensible and convenient once the patient is happy with the medication and well controlled, provided there are no major cost implications. Beware of unfamiliar drug combinations that may contain the same class of drug as already being prescribed singly. The Prodigy guideline on hypertension contains detailed lists of recommended medication for treatment of hypertension.[10]

Special groups of patients

Ethnic groups

Patients of Asian origin with hypertension are more at risk of diabetes and coronary artery disease. Use thiazides with caution as they can worsen glucose intolerance. Patients of Afro-Caribbean origin seem to respond less well to beta-blockers and ACE inhibitors and you will achieve better control on thiazide and calcium channel antagonists.[11]

Older people with hypertension

Hypertension, especially isolated systolic hypertension (160 mmHg systolic with a diastolic of less than 90 mmHg) is found in more than half of those over 60 years. Over-60 year olds with hypertension have a higher risk of cardiovascular complications than younger people. Women over the age of 70 years have a higher risk of cardiovascular disease, particularly of stroke, than men of that age. Treatment, continued to at least the age of 80 years, has been shown to reduce the risks of cardiovascular disease.[2] Thiazides are the first choice for drug treatment or dihydropyridine calcium antagonists if thiazides are contraindicated, not tolerated or are ineffective.

Patients with diabetes

The studies of people with type 2 diabetes looked at cardiovascular events as secondary events, rather than the main endpoints. However, comparative trials suggest that ACE inhibitors are better than calcium channel antagonists in preventing cardiovascular events. As far as possible levels of blood pressure in people with diabetes should be controlled to below 140/80 mmHg. The Heart Outcomes Prevention Evaluation (HOPE) trial found that there were significantly fewer diabetic complications – diabetic nephropathy and retinopathy – among patients with diabetes who took ramipril.[12] The beneficial effects could not be attributed to the effects of blood pressure reduction alone, as the overall reduction was only 2–3 mmHg. Most patients with diabetes (about 80%) would qualify for treatment with ramipril if you accept the conclusions of the HOPE trial. This has obvious implications for drug budgets, but could reduce the overall cost of complications of diabetes as well as providing considerable health gain.

Malignant hypertension

This is an emergency, fortunately rare, with a very poor outcome if left untreated. Even when treated, a high proportion go on to develop strokes or renal failure. The diagnostic criteria are a diastolic blood pressure of over 120 mmHg together with advanced hypertensive retinopathy (haemorrhages and exudates, with or without papilloedema). It is more common in smokers and people of Afro-Caribbean origin. Recommended treatment includes a reduction in blood pressure over about one week (to avoid precipitating a stroke by too rapid a reduction). You will probably want to seek specialist help especially as secondary hypertension is more common in this group than in those with non-malignant hypertension, and patients will require investigation to exclude a precipitating cause.

Follow up

The frequency of follow-up visits will depend on Mr Round's overall risk category, as well as on the level of blood pressure. Once the target level of blood pressure has been reached and other risk factors have been controlled or excluded, agree what the follow-up regime should be. Some patients are happy to monitor their own blood pressure at home (with a suitable machine) and can be seen less often. If Mr Round expresses undue anxiety about lengthening the interval between checks to six-monthly, this is an opportunity to correct any misconceptions about the aims of treatment.

It is important that patients not on drug treatment understand the need for monitoring and follow up and for periodic reconsideration of the need for drug treatment.

In more complex cases, patients should be seen at more frequent intervals. If the therapeutic goals, including the control of blood pressure, have not been reached within six months, consider referral to a specialist in hypertension.

Antihypertensive therapy is generally for life. Stopping treatment in patients who have been correctly diagnosed as hypertensive is usually followed, sooner or later, by the return of blood pressure to pretreatment levels. Nevertheless, after prolonged blood pressure control, you may be able to gradually reduce the dose or number of drugs used, particularly among patients who have made great strides in observing lifestyle (non-drug) measures. Keep monitoring carefully to ensure that levels do not climb steadily upwards with a reduction in medication, or with an increase in weight with increasing age. Remain alert to any incipient additional risk factors.

Quality indicators in hypertension

Hypertension is included in the targets for quality indicators because of its importance in the prevention of coronary heart disease, heart failure and stroke. The quality points available are achievable on a sliding scale, so as you are collecting the data to demonstrate your own competence you are also helping to show that your practice is achieving high standards of care. A total of 105 points is available for hypertension management. A further 53 points can be found in the management of blood pressure in the diabetes, coronary heart disease and stroke indicator sets. Organisational points for screening the practice population for hypertension add another 15 points. Domains for recording and checking with audits include:

- 55% of patients over 45 years of age screened for hypertension: 10 points
- 75% of patients over 45 years of age screened for hypertension: 15 points
- a register of all patients with a blood pressure over a systolic of 160 mmHg and a diastolic of 100 mmHg measured according to the British Hypertension Society Guidelines (*see* Chapter 4): 9 points[2]
- 90% of all patients on the hypertension register have had their smoking status recorded: 10 points
- 90% of those on the hypertension register recorded as smokers have been offered smoking cessation advice: 10 points
- 90% of patients on the hypertension register have had a blood pressure measurement in the last nine months: 20 points

- 70% of patients on the hypertension register have a blood pressure on treatment of less than that recommended by the British Hypertension Society Guidelines (150/90 mmHg): 56 points.[2]

Patients can be excluded from these targets if they:

- refuse, or fail to attend, at least three invitations in the last 12 months
- refuse to allow their blood pressure to be measured
- have a condition that renders hypertension management irrelevant e.g. in the terminally ill
- cannot tolerate, or have contraindications to, medication to control the hypertension
- have been diagnosed with hypertension for less than nine months.

Collecting data to demonstrate your learning, competence, performance and standards of service delivery

Example cycle of evidence 5.1

- Focus: keeping up to date
- Other relevant focus: relationships with patients

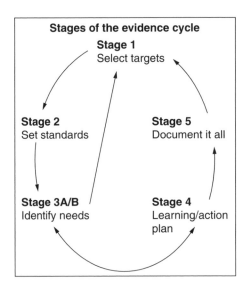

Stages of the evidence cycle

Stage 1
Select targets

Stage 2
Set standards

Stage 5
Document it all

Stage 3A/B
Identify needs

Stage 4
Learning/action plan

> **Box 5.2:**   Case study
>
> Mr Director attends for a review of his medication and hypertension. He was asked to make an appointment with the practice nurse but he comes to see you instead. He brings with him a printout from the Internet and says that he would like to change his medication. He has been on a thiazide diuretic and a beta-blocker for about 12 years, and has read that these drugs increase his lipid levels. The Internet article says that he should be lowering his cholesterol whatever his level (you have previously assured him that his is normal) and is asking for a 'new drug' – an angiotension-receptor blocker.

This is just an example. Keep your task simple. You could choose three or four cycles of evidence to demonstrate your competence each year.

Stage 1: Select your aspirations for good practice

The excellent GP:

- provides or arranges investigations or treatment when necessary
- does not allow his or her beliefs to influence the advice or treatment provided, or if their beliefs are likely to affect patient management tells patients of their right to see another doctor
- refers to another practitioner when indicated.

Stage 2: Set the standards for your outcomes

Outcomes might include:

- the way learning is applied
- a learnt skill
- a protocol
- a strategy that is implemented
- meeting recommended standards.

- Demonstrate consistent best practice in managing hypertension in line with current guidelines.
- Make efficient use of resources.
- Empower patients to take decisions about their management.

Stage 3A: Identify your learning needs

- Self-assess your knowledge about current guidelines for the management of hypertension.
- Use a significant event audit e.g. a patient who suffered a stroke despite attending regularly for review of his hypertension.
- Use your reflective diary to capture trends or comments relating to problems dealing with patients who bring information culled from the Internet or other publications.
- Reflect on your previous advice that a normal cholesterol level does not require action in someone with hypertension.

Stage 3B: Identify your service needs

Any of the needs assessment exercises in 3A may also reveal service needs.

- Record the pathway of care when patients with hypertension are reviewed and identify any gaps or overlaps.
- Identify and review the guidelines for hypertension management used in the practice to determine if they are still appropriate in view of recent publications.
- Collect data about access and arrangements for referral to specialists in hypertension management.

Stage 4: Make and carry out a learning and action plan

- Compare your knowledge of the investigation and management of hypertension with an authoritative source you obtain and read.
- Prepare a draft revision of the practice guidelines for the investigation and management of hypertension.
- Arrange a presentation of your new knowledge and discuss your draft revised guidelines at a practice meeting.
- Discuss with other health professionals how they manage patients who bring information culled from the Internet or other media.

Stage 5: Document your learning, competence, performance and standards of service delivery

- Collect feedback from other health professionals about your draft guidelines for the investigation and management of hypertension.

- Keep the revised guidelines for management of hypertension.
- Record extracts of information from your reflective diary about your greater understanding of how you manage the situation when patients bring in information from other sources, and the changes you have made so that you feel that your attitude is not perceived as dismissive or defensive.

Box 5.3:   Case study continued

You ask Mr Director if you can study the information that he has and get in touch with him when you have obtained sufficient information yourself to be able to have an informed discussion of the options. Once you have all the facts you set aside a longer appointment time and go through all the evidence with him. You agree together that he will try a traditional ACE inhibitor first to see if this will control his hypertension as well as it has been in the past. If he has an ACE inhibitor-provoked cough (or any deterioration of his renal function), you will discuss other changes in treatment with him in the future.

Example cycle of evidence 5.2

- Focus: working with colleagues
- Other relevant foci: maintaining good medical practice; teaching and training

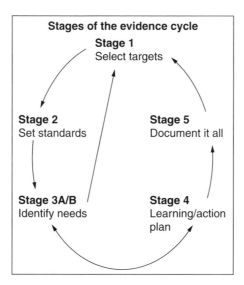

Stages of the evidence cycle

Stage 1
Select targets

Stage 2
Set standards

Stage 5
Document it all

Stage 3A/B
Identify needs

Stage 4
Learning/action plan

Box 5.4:   Case study

You are consulting in parallel with the new practice nurse reviewing patients with hypertension, to ensure that the practice meets the quality framework requirements. She has recently done the practice nurse training after working as a specialist nurse in a cardiology unit. She complains to you that she had difficulty finding a working blood pressure machine. The machine in her treatment room had leaky connections and she had to borrow a large cuff from one of the consulting rooms. She asks if you will help her move the desk in her room before the next patient is seen. The chair cannot be placed next to the desk and she cannot support the arm at heart level. She also queries the protocol as it only calls for one sitting blood pressure reading to be taken. She is used to doing two readings and doing a standing reading in patients over the age of 65 years.

This is just an example. Keep your task simple. You could choose three or four cycles of evidence to demonstrate your competence each year.

Stage 1: Select your aspirations for good practice

The excellent GP:

- respects the skills and contributions of colleagues
- helps to educate other colleagues at all levels
- joins in with reviews and audits of standards and performance of the team, and with any steps to remedy deficiencies.

Stage 2: Set the standards for your outcomes

Outcomes might include:

- the way learning is applied
- a learnt skill
- a protocol
- a strategy that is implemented
- meeting recommended standards.

- Demonstrate that blood pressure measurement is carried out in line with best practice.[13]

- The practice protocol for reviewing patients with hypertension is in line with best practice.

Stage 3A: Identify your learning needs

- Compare your awareness of the causes of error in measuring blood pressure with an authoritative source.[2,14]
- Self-assess your own technique of measuring blood pressure.
- Check that your knowledge about hypertension measurement is up to date.
- Record your observations in your reflective diary about how you manage the challenge of implied criticism from a new employee.

Stage 3B: Identify your service needs

Any of the needs assessment exercises in 3A may also reveal service needs.

- Ask the practice manager to arrange for a review of the condition and availability of all the blood pressure equipment in the practice.
- Audit the skills of all staff who take blood pressures with a self-assessment checklist of how they take blood pressures.[13]

Stage 4: Make and carry out a learning and action plan

- Arrange a practice meeting to discuss the audit on avoiding sources of error when recording blood pressure and agree the necessary changes.
- Obtain a poster on how to take blood pressure to display in the treatment room.
- Set up with the practice manager a computer recall system for regular maintenance of blood pressure equipment and a supply of spare machines and cuffs.
- Revise the practice protocol for blood pressure reviews in the light of up-to-date recommendations.

Stage 5: Document your learning, competence, performance and standards of service delivery

- Repeat the audit of avoidance of errors when recording blood pressure after the necessary changes have been made.
- Review the condition of blood pressure measuring equipment in 12 months.

- Produce a revised protocol which is available to all staff on a link from all computer screens and on a laminated sheet for those who prefer written materials.

Box 5.5: Case study continued

After six months, you are able to leave most of the management of hypertension reviews to the practice nurse. She learns how to make attractive charts of how everyone is doing from data collected into an Excel computer package and the GPs thank her for her contribution to maximising the number of quality points the practice is achieving.

Example cycle of evidence 5.3

- Focus: research
- Other relevant foci: probity; relationships with patients

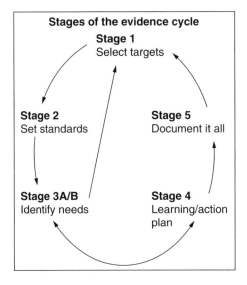

Stages of the evidence cycle

Stage 1
Select targets

Stage 2
Set standards

Stage 5
Document it all

Stage 3A/B
Identify needs

Stage 4
Learning/action plan

> **Box 5.6:** Case study
>
> A pharmaceutical representative approaches Dr Tempted after he chaired a meeting on modern methods of treating hypertension. The representative asks if he will carry out some post-marketing research for the company. The company will supply all the paperwork and a 24-hour blood pressure monitor, which the practice can keep at the end of the study. Dr Tempted just has to find at least 20 patients with poorly controlled blood pressure – that should be easy, he thinks – and enrol them into the study. The patients have a 24-hour recording before, and eight weeks after, adding an extra pill to their regime. The patients are asked to fill in a diary of symptoms before and after the additional medication. If the blood pressure is better controlled, the company will provide supplies of the medication for the period of the study. Then Dr Tempted can continue the medication by prescribing it, as it is already released onto the market.

This is just an example. Keep your task simple. You could choose three or four cycles of evidence to demonstrate your competence each year.

Stage 1: Select your aspirations for good practice

The excellent GP:

- puts the care and safety of patients first when participating in research
- ensures that approval has been obtained for research from an independent research ethics committee and that patients have given informed consent
- uses resources wisely
- ensures that his or her financial affairs are capable of withstanding searching external audit.

Stage 2: Set the standards for your outcomes

> Outcomes might include:
>
> - the way learning is applied
> - a learnt skill
> - a protocol
> - a strategy that is implemented
> - meeting recommended standards.

- Show that research is carried out in an ethical manner with honesty and integrity.

Stage 3A: Identify your learning needs

- Obtain and read through the documentation supplied by the pharmaceutical company and compare the ethical considerations with a reference document on the ethics of post-marketing surveillance. You might look at www.mrc.ac.uk/pdf-peer_review.pdf or www.wellcome.ac.uk/en/1/awtvispolgrpgid.html for a checklist of questions to ask.
- Compare the characteristics of the proposed medication, the contraindications and possible side-effects with the patient information supplied.

Stage 3B: Identify your service needs

> Any of the needs assessment exercises in 3A may also reveal service needs.

- Review with the practice and with the medicines manager of your PCO whether the proposed medication is one likely to be approved for use in your area, or whether the cost-effectiveness is less than a similar preparation.

Stage 4: Make and carry out a learning and action plan

- Present a summary of the proposals at a practice meeting for discussion with your peers.
- Look up the characteristics of the proposed medication, the contraindications and possible side-effects. Compare this with the patient information supplied. You might consult a source on patient information such as www.esds.ac.uk/qualidata/create/furtherreading.asp.
- Prepare a cost-effectiveness analysis of the preparation to be used in the study, and, if required, resolve to discuss with all patients involved changing onto a similar but more cost-effective preparation at the end of the study.
- Carry out the study and ensure that all the paperwork is completed correctly before submission.

Stage 5: Document your learning, competence, performance and standards of service delivery

- Keep a duplicate record of the paperwork and your results.
- Record the gift of the 24-hour blood pressure monitor at the end of the study in the practice newsletter and thank all the patients for their participation.
- Record the number of patients who agreed to change medication to a more cost-effective similar preparation at the end of the study.

Box 5.7:   Case study continued

Dr Tempted discussed the study with his PCO and entered the research on their register. The medication supplied by the pharmaceutical company was considerably more expensive than an equivalent medication in the same group. He agreed with the pharmaceutical adviser to the PCO that he would offer those patients who required additional medication an opportunity to change onto a more cost-effective medication with informed consent at the end of the study.

Dr Tempted completed the study according to the protocol supplied by the pharmaceutical company. Then he presented the cost-effectiveness data to the patients who had required the additional medication. He found that they were all willing to co-operate with his desire not to involve the health service in excess expenditure, and were willing to change onto the lower cost equivalent. He was able to record that he had successfully resisted the temptation to use a drug he would not otherwise have used, in order to obtain a desired piece of equipment for the practice.

References

1   Fahey TP and Peters TJ (1996) What constitutes controlled hypertension? Patient based comparison of hypertension guidelines. *British Medical Journal.* **313**: 93–6.

2   Ramsay LE, Williams B, Johnston GD *et al.* (1999) British Hypertension Society Guidelines for hypertension management 1999: summary. *British Medical Journal.* **319**: 630–5.

3   NHS Executive (2000) *National Service Framework for Coronary Heart Disease.* Department of Health, London.

4   Anderson OK, Almgreen T, Persoson B *et al.* (1998) Survival after treated hypertension. *British Medical Journal.* **317**: 167–71.

5   Foord-Kelcey G (ed.) (2003) *Guidelines* vol. 20. Medendium Group Publishing Ltd, Berkhamsted.

6   www.eguidelines.co.uk.

7   Guidelines Committee (2003) European Society of Hypertension – European Society of Cardiology guidelines for the management of arterial hypertension (2003). *Journal of Hypertension.* **21(6)**: 1011–53.

8   Godlee F (ed.) (2003) *Clinical Evidence.* BMJ Publishing Group, London. www.clinicalevidence.com.

9   Hansson L, Zanchetti A, Carruthers SG *et al.*, for the HOT Study Group (1998) Effects of intensive blood-pressure lowering and low-dose aspirin in patients with hypertension: principal results of the Hypertension Optimal Treatment (HOT) randomized trial. *Lancet.* **351**: 1755–62.

10   www.prodigy.nhs.uk.

11   Lip GYH, O'Brien E and Beevers G (eds) (2000) *ABC of Hypertension* (4e). BMJ Publications, London.

12   The Heart Outcomes Prevention Evaluation (HOPE) Investigators (2000) Effects of an angiotensin-converting enzyme inhibitor, ramipril, on cardiovascular events in high risk patients. *New England Journal of Medicine.* **342**: 1445–53.

13   Chambers R, Wakley G and Iqbal Z (2001) *Cardiovascular Matters in Primary Care.* Radcliffe Medical Press, Oxford.

14   Dillon M, Littler WA, Mee F *et al.* (1997) *Recommendations on Blood Pressure Measurement* (2e). BMJ Books, London.

6

Heart failure

> **Box 6.1:** Case study
>
> Mr Marrow grumbles as you check his blood pressure, 'I'm getting old, doc, I'll have to give up the gardening, can't do it any more'. He tells you that he is getting out of breath when he works in the garden and has developed an irritating cough, especially when he wakes in the night and in the morning. He had an admission to hospital six years ago with a myocardial infarction and has been taking aspirin, a beta-blocker, a statin and an ACE inhibitor since. He has not smoked since the shock of being admitted to hospital with chest pain, as his father and his elder brother both died from heart attacks. Although over-weight with a BMI of 30, he has always been a keen gardener, growing much of his own food, especially since his retirement. He is now aged 68 years. On further enquiry, he has noticed the tops of his socks leave a dent all round his ankles by the end of the day, but he sleeps on two pillows – always has done – and there is no change in his appetite or bowels. He takes occasional courses of a non-steroidal anti-inflammatory drug when he has overdone things in the garden.

What issues you should cover

Exercise-induced ventricular dysfunction, usually due to myocardial ischaemia, may cause a rise in ventricular filling pressure and a fall in cardiac output and induce symptoms of heart failure such as breathlessness. However, as both the underlying causes and the treatment of this condition are generally differ-ent from those of heart failure secondary to chronic ventricular dysfunction, such patients should not be diagnosed as having chronic heart failure.

Consider heart failure at an early stage

Congestive heart failure is the failure of the heart muscle to pump enough blood to meet the body's needs. When the heart muscle pump cannot handle the amount of blood it gets, the blood slows down and backs up. This puts pres-sure on the blood vessels in the lungs, legs and abdomen and causes leakage from these blood vessels so that fluid collects in the tissues. The heart chambers get bigger (cardiomegaly) over time to decrease the backup. Although this helps in the early stages, it makes the heart pump less well in the long run.

The causes of heart failure include:

- coronary artery disease (the commonest cause)
- hypertension
- valvular disease
- cor pulmonale (causing right-sided ventricular failure)
- cardiomyopathy
- drugs including alcohol.

Symptoms and signs

Heart muscle weakness can occur in one or both of the ventricles. In left-sided failure, the decreased flow to the kidneys triggers off antidiuretic hormone production leading to retention of fluid and sodium and can result in a sudden increase in weight. The pressure in the left atrium and in the lungs also increases. Typical symptoms are shortness of breath, an irritating cough with white sputum, waking up breathless at night and having to sleep propped up on pillows or in a chair. If the right side of the heart is affected, symptoms may include ankle oedema, upper abdominal tenderness with a bloated discomfort, a lack of appetite and fatigue. Misdiagnosis is common, due either to missing the condition or labelling other conditions as heart failure (*see* Box 6.2).

Box 6.2:   Other conditions with similar symptoms to heart failure[1]

Chronic chest diseases	Pulmonary embolic disease
Venous insufficiency in the lower limbs	Severe anaemia
Thyroid disease	Renal or hepatic disease
Drug-induced fluid retention e.g. from non-steroidal anti-inflammatory drugs	Drug-induced ankle swelling e.g. from calcium channel blockers
Obesity	Low albumin levels
Bilateral renal artery stenosis	Depression and/or anxiety disorders

---

Take a careful history from Mr Marrow as the history will often lead you towards the diagnosis and the cause. The most specific signs you might find on examination are a raised jugular venous pressure and a displaced apex beat – but Mr Marrow may have neither of these and still have heart failure.

Crackles at the lung bases, an enlarged tender liver, peripheral oedema and third or fourth heart sounds are not specific and may be found in other conditions.

The severity of heart failure is graded according to the New York Association classification of heart failure symptoms. This classification appears in the SIGN guidelines:[2]

- Class I: no limitation, ordinary exercise does not cause symptoms
- Class II: slight limitation of physical activity
- Class III: marked limitation of physical activity
- Class IV: inability to engage in any physical activity without discomfort.

Investigations

Both the guidelines from NICE and the National Service Framework for coronary heart disease recommend that heart failure should be a diagnosis that is positively confirmed.[1,3]

Investigations are needed to:

- confirm or refute the diagnosis of heart failure
- define the underlying cause if possible
- identify factors that may make it worse or better
- help with the decisions about managing the condition
- provide a baseline for monitoring the condition
- make a prognosis for the future.

You may want to do some routine blood tests on Mr Marrow, mostly to exclude other causes for the symptoms or to provide a baseline for monitoring treatment. These include urea, electrolytes and creatinine, full blood count, thyroid function and liver function tests, a fasting glucose and lipid profile. You might want to arrange for a chest X-ray, peak flow rate, spirometry, and test the urine for albumin. A chest X-ray may show cardiac enlargement, pulmonary venous congestion or pulmonary oedema, but is of limited value as significant left ventricular dysfunction may be present without cardiomegaly. The chest X-ray, peak flow or spirometry may reveal alternative reasons for breathlessness.

A 12-lead ECG will usually confirm or refute the diagnosis of heart failure. Natriuretic peptides – B-type natriuretic peptide (BNP) or N-terminal pro-B-type natriuretic peptide (NTproBNP) – should also be tested if this is possible at your laboratory. If both these tests are normal then heart failure is unlikely. If one or both are abnormal, then arrange echocardiography.

You may have a local echocardiography service with a GPwSI in echocardiography, or be interested in providing this yourself. The competencies required are to undertake echocardiograms to levels of peer accuracy with patient comfort and satisfaction, while maintaining patient safety. The GP should be competent to undertake and report on adult echocardiography. The GP must be able to work as a team member in the local service, collaborate with the PCO(s), acute trust(s) and the lead in service development, and offer education to local GPs to improve appropriateness of use of the service. You can look at the recommendations for a GP led service on the Internet.[4]

Echocardiography using reflected ultrasound can be used to:

- provide an accurate assessment of left ventricular function
- demonstrate features suggestive of diastolic dysfunction
- show any structural abnormalities that might be responsible for heart failure
- assess the significance of heart murmurs
- screen healthy people who have a family history of cardiomyopathy.

If echocardiography is normal, then chronic heart failure is unlikely. Refer for a specialist opinion if you are still doubtful.

If a poor picture is obtained with echocardiography, then radionuclide angiography, cardiac magnetic resonance or transoesophageal Doppler 2D echocardiography may be arranged by secondary care. Even these investigations may occasionally not give a clear diagnosis, or may continue to suggest diastolic heart failure, so that you will need to seek specialist advice.

Treatment options[1-3]

Active treatment for heart failure can postpone progression to more severe symptoms. Unfortunately, most patients with heart failure are elderly and suffer from other conditions requiring multiple medications. You need to review the multiple medications and stop any that are not giving a clear benefit.[5]

General lifestyle advice

You will have given much of this advice previously to patients who have the underlying causes of heart failure listed above. It is worth reinforcing the advice and going through the benefits that can be achieved:

- take regular aerobic and/or resistive exercise. Enrolling on a tailored exercise programme could help
- stop smoking. Patients may be helped with support from a smoking cessation service
- reduce salt intake. Give advice about salt substitutes as most of these contain potassium. Excess use of potassium may cause problems when using ACE inhibitors or potassium-sparing diuretics

- alcohol is contraindicated in alcohol-induced cardiomyopathy, but otherwise may be helpful in small quantities of one to two units daily.[1] Tailor your advice to the patient e.g. someone who needs to lose weight may need to avoid alcohol as part of their calorie reduction
- advise gradual weight loss in those whose BMI is above the desirable range
- sexual activity may need to be tailored to the degree of breathlessness. Advice on a less active role and modifications of technique can help people to feel less anxious about continuing sexual activity
- air travel is possible for the majority of people with heart failure, but give advice about sitting in an aisle seat so people can easily visit the toilet and keep active.

Diuretics

Use diuretics to relieve fluid retention and congestion. A loop diuretic is the mainstay of treatment e.g. furosemide (frusemide), bumetanide or torasemide. Adding a thiazide may promote a dramatic diuresis, so that close and frequent monitoring of electrolytes and fluid balance is needed. If you prescribe potassium-sparing diuretics, e.g. amiloride, triampterene, carry out careful electrolyte monitoring in patients who are on ACE inhibitors, in case potassium levels rise to dangerous levels.

Gout can be made worse by diuretics and non-steroidal anti-inflammatory drugs will worsen fluid retention. Colchicine is useful if an acute attack of gout is precipitated. Consider adding low dose spironolactone (12.5–50 mg daily) to other medications in patients who have Class III or IV degrees of heart failure despite adequate treatment. You may want to seek specialist advice, as well as carefully monitoring biochemical parameters.

Angiotensin converting enzyme inhibitors

All patients with symptoms or evidence of heart failure should be treated with an ACE inhibitor. Explain to patients that treatment delays the development of more severe symptoms, reduces cardiovascular events and increases survival. There is no good evidence of differences between the various ACE inhibitor drugs, so choose the cheapest and best tolerated one.

ACE inhibitors may cause deterioration of renal function, so check that serum creatinine levels are not raised before treatment and after each increase of dose. If the serum creatinine is more than 200 mmol/litre, refer for specialist advice before starting treatment.

Start with a low dose and increase by doubling the dose at not less than two-week intervals. Aim at the target dose recommended by the manufacturer, or at the maximum tolerated dose. Monitor the electrolytes (particularly potassium), urea, creatinine and blood pressure.

If the patient develops low blood pressure with no symptoms continue at that dose. However, if the patient complains of dizziness, feeling light-headed and/or confused you may need to adjust or stop other medication such as nitrates or other vasodilators. Stop calcium channel blockers unless they are essential for angina or hypertension. You may be able to reduce diuretic dosage if the patient has no signs of congestion.

Cough is common in chronic heart failure and many sufferers have chronic lung disease as well. Cough may be a symptom of pulmonary oedema. If cough has increased since the introduction of ACE inhibitor therapy and is interfering with sleep, try an angiotensin II receptor antagonist instead.

If urea, creatinine or potassium rise excessively, check what other medication the patient is taking (including non-prescribed agents). If possible, stop any nephrotoxic drugs e.g. non-steroidal anti-inflammatory drugs (NSAIDs), non-essential vasodilators e.g. nitrates or calcium antagonists and potassium-retaining diuretics. Reduce loop diuretics if no pulmonary congestion is present. If this does not result in better biochemical parameters, halve the dose of the ACE inhibitor and recheck. If you still have problems, ask for specialist help.

Angiotensin II receptor antagonists

These drugs are not licensed for the treatment of chronic heart failure, but evidence is accumulating that they should be at least as effective as ACE inhibitors and may be useful in addition.[6,7]

Beta-blocker drugs

These drugs are licensed for treatment of heart failure and adding them to standard treatment with ACE inhibitors in patients with mild to moderate heart failure (Class I, II or III) reduces hospital admissions for increased symptoms and the risk of death. Many doctors are nervous about adding this type of drug, as for many years the advice given was to avoid beta-blockers in heart failure. Start bisoprolol or carvedilol (the two licensed drugs) at a low dose and gradually titrate upwards. Very close monitoring is needed – at least every two weeks – and patients should weigh themselves daily for any persistent weight gain that might signal increased fluid retention.

Do not use beta-blockers in patients who have reversible airways disease.

Patients need to be aware that symptomatic improvement is slow over three to six months or longer, and that symptomatic deterioration occurs in about one-fifth to one-third of patients during the titration period. Tiredness, fatigue and breathlessness can usually be controlled by adjustments to other medication:

- if congestion increases, the dose of diuretic can be doubled and/or the dose of the beta-blocker halved

- if fatigue is too great, halve the dose
- if the pulse rate is less than 50/minute and there are worsening symptoms, halve the dose, or, rarely, stop the beta-blocker. Do not stop a beta-blocker suddenly as there is a risk of a rebound increase in myocardial ischaemia or infarction. Seek specialist advice first. Discontinue any other rate-limiting drugs unless they are essential e.g. digoxin, amiodarone, diltiazem. Rule out heart block with an ECG
- if the patient develops low blood pressure but has no symptoms continue at that dose. However, if the patient complains of dizziness, feeling light-headed and/or confused you may need to adjust or stop other medication such as nitrates or other vasodilators. Stop calcium channel blockers unless they are absolutely essential for angina or hypertension. You may be able to reduce diuretic dosage if the patient has no signs of congestion.

Digoxin

In patients who are already taking diuretics and ACE inhibitors, digoxin decreases the rate of admissions to hospital for worsening symptoms. Patients may also need digoxin if they have atrial fibrillation and heart failure.

Calcium channel blockers

Amlodipine can be used for patients with hypertension and/or angina, but other agents e.g. verapamil, diltiazem, from this group of drugs should be avoided.

Aspirin and statins in patients with underlying arteriosclerotic disease

Most patients with arteriosclerotic disease, including coronary artery disease, will already be taking aspirin and this should be continued if they develop heart failure. Similarly, if statins are indicated they should be continued.

Specialist initiation of treatment

Take advice from a specialist before prescribing amiodarone. Review side-effects together with liver and thyroid function every six months.

Anticoagulants are used when patients have atrial fibrillation, or for those with a history of thromboembolism, left ventricular aneurysm or intracardiac thrombosis. Arrangements for regular monitoring must be clear to both patients and health professionals. Too often, the patient is unaware when the next test should be done or there is confusion about where the blood test will be taken. Make clear arrangements about how to let patients know safely about what dose they should be taking. Think about how they will manage if complex instructions are given, such as 'four milligrams and three milligrams on alternate days'. It is very difficult to take different doses on alternate days unless you are very organised.

Isosorbide with hydralazine combination treatment can be used in patients who are intolerant of ACE inhibitors or angiotensin II receptor antagonists.

Intravenous inotropic agents are usually only used short-term for acute exacerbations of heart failure.

Monitoring heart failure

The interval between clinical reviews depends on the response to treatment and the incidence of symptoms. Most patients with heart failure have multiple medical conditions, so you are likely to be seeing them frequently. It is easy to get so involved with the management of each individual condition that you may have difficulty remembering to do routine checks like electrolytes and creatinine. Set up a reminder system, so that you do not have to check when the blood tests, weight and blood pressure measurements are due every time the patient attends.

Quality indicators in heart failure

The quality points available are achievable on a sliding scale, so as you are collecting the data to demonstrate your own competence you are also helping to show that your practice is achieving high standards of care. Those patients who have left ventricular dysfunction have additional quality points to those applicable for coronary heart disease:

- a register of patients with left ventricular dysfunction: 4 points
- 90% of patients on the register have the diagnosis (made after 1 April 2003) confirmed by echocardiogram: 6 points
- 70% of patients on the register are currently on an ACE inhibitor or an angiotensin II antagonist: 10 points.

Exception reporting will be the same as for the quality targets for hypertension. That is, if the patients do not wish to participate, have contraindications or unacceptable side-effects on medication, or have conditions making treatment inappropriate.

Collecting data to demonstrate your learning, competence, performance and standards of service delivery

Example cycle of evidence 6.1

- Focus: good medical practice
- Other relevant foci: relationships with patients; working with colleagues

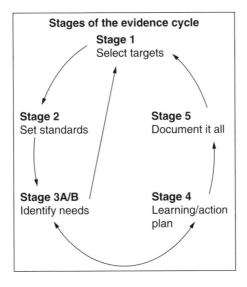

Stages of the evidence cycle

Stage 1
Select targets

Stage 2
Set standards

Stage 5
Document it all

Stage 3A/B
Identify needs

Stage 4
Learning/action plan

Box 6.3: Case study

You have recently joined a general practice and have volunteered to 'clean up the data' relating to the diagnosis of heart failure. As you go through the records of patients with a Read coding for heart failure, you find that many of them have not had their diagnosis confirmed. You want to recall these patients but do not want to alarm them, or upset any of your colleagues who have been responsible for their care. You are concerned to find that the waiting time for echocardiography is seven months.

This is just an example. Keep your task simple. You could choose three or four cycles of evidence to demonstrate your competence each year.

Stage 1: Select your aspirations for good practice

The excellent GP:

- is competent when making a diagnosis and giving or arranging treatment
- provides or arranges investigations or treatment when necessary
- makes efficient use of resources, but records, reports and endeavours to rectify deficiencies in resources
- consults with colleagues and keeps them informed when sharing the care of patients
- empowers patients to take decisions about their management
- can justify claiming quality points for heart failure care.

Stage 2: Set the standards for your outcomes

Outcomes might include:

- the way learning is applied
- a learnt skill
- a protocol
- a strategy that is implemented
- meeting recommended standards.

- Demonstrate consistent best practice in the diagnosis and treatment of heart failure.
- Be able to substantiate claims for quality.

Stage 3A: Identify your learning needs

- Self-assess your knowledge about the guidelines for management of heart failure.
- Carry out a significant event audit e.g. a patient with heart failure who required admission for deteriorating renal function having not had a creatinine measurement for two years.
- Use your reflective diary to capture trends or comments relating to problems dealing with your colleagues who are feeling criticised by your enthusiasm for evidence-based medicine.
- Identify methods of collecting feedback from patients without adding to their burdens.

Stage 3B: Identify your service needs

> Any of the needs assessment exercises in 3A may also reveal service needs.

- Audit how patients on diuretics and ACE inhibitors are monitored, e.g. on a sample of 20 patients.
- Collect data about access and arrangements for referral for echocardiography.

Stage 4: Make and carry out a learning and action plan

- Compare your knowledge of the investigation and management of heart failure with the NICE guidelines.[1]
- Prepare and run an in-house multidisciplinary discussion group on the implementation of the NICE guidelines for heart failure.
- Set up an audit of the monitoring of patients with heart failure who are on diuretics and ACE inhibitors, and record what changes you think should be made. Present this at a practice meeting.
- Capture patient comments about the way in which they have been recalled for review of their diagnosis.
- Obtain statistics about the workload and waiting times for echocardiography and how you can make representations to try to improve the availability of services.

Stage 5: Document your learning, competence, performance and standards of service delivery

- Record the way in which the practice will implement the NICE guidelines on heart failure and the comments from your colleagues about the advantages and difficulties.[1]
- Keep the audit of the monitoring of patients with heart failure who are on diuretics and ACE inhibitors and the changes agreed, and schedule a repeat audit in 12 months' time.
- Keep extracts of information from your reflective diary about your greater understanding of your colleagues' objections to your enthusiasm for evidence-based care.
- Record patients' comments about the way in which they have been recalled for review of their diagnosis. Add your reflections about any changes that you need to make if you repeat the exercise for another disease.
- Keep feedback from the representations you have made about the availability of echocardiography.

Box 6.4:   Case study continued

You draw up a list of patients needing review to confirm their diagnosis. You arrange with your partners which patients they want to see and which ones you can review. Over the next nine months, all of the patients on the list are reviewed and some are referred for echocardiography. You add a reminder flag so that each time a patient with heart failure who is on diuretics or an ACE inhibitor has the results of a blood test entered on their record, an automatic reminder is generated for when another test should be done. Most patients seem to be pleased with the extra attention they are receiving, but a few seem disgruntled at having to make changes to their treatment. You were told by your PCO that extra provision for echocardiography was already in the pipeline for this financial year.

Example cycle of evidence 6.2

- Focus: relationships with patients
- Other relevant focus: working with colleagues

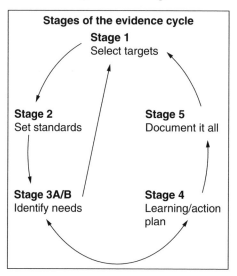

Stages of the evidence cycle

Stage 1
Select targets

Stage 2
Set standards

Stage 5
Document it all

Stage 3A/B
Identify needs

Stage 4
Learning/action plan

Box 6.5:   Case study

Mrs Shelter's daughter asks for her mother to be registered at the practice and this is arranged. Mrs Shelter is brought in to see the practice nurse two days later for her 'new patient medical'. The practice nurse comes to see you about her, as she is worried about her management. Mrs Shelter has recently been

continued opposite

discharged from hospital in another part of the country and has moved to live with her daughter. She has a long list of medications, but neither she, nor her daughter, are clear how they should be taken, or what they are for. When you see her, it looks to you as if she has had a diagnosis of chronic heart failure made. You can tell her how to take her medication, but you decide to contact the hospital from which she was discharged for some information. You also arrange some blood tests.

This is just an example. Keep your task simple. You could choose three or four cycles of evidence to demonstrate your competence each year.

Stage 1: Select your aspirations for good practice

The excellent GP:

- gives patients the information they need about their problem in a way they can understand
- empowers patients to take decisions about their management
- resists the temptation to appear superior by denigrating the care patients have received from others.

Stage 2: Set the standards for your outcomes

Outcomes might include:

- the way learning is applied
- a learnt skill
- a protocol
- a strategy that is implemented
- meeting recommended standards.

- Patients with heart failure receive a copy of the version of the NICE guidelines written for patients, their carers and the public.
- A management plan is received within 48 hours from the hospital discharging the patient, and the patient and carer are aware of its content.

Stage 3A: Identify your learning needs

- Compare your management of heart failure with the NICE guidelines for any gaps in your knowledge.[1]
- Audit the proportion of your patients with chronic heart failure (and/or their carers) who know that they have a management plan when discharged from hospital.
- Record in your reflective diary how you explain to patients about failures in communication between hospital and general practice.

Stage 3B: Identify your service needs

> Any of the needs assessment exercises in 3A may also reveal service needs.

- Identify if you have a supply of patient versions of the NICE guidelines on chronic heart failure.
- Undertake a significant event audit with key members of the practice team of e.g. a patient whose medication was incorrectly issued because the information in the discharge letter he brought in from the hospital was not acted upon.
- Ask the practice manager to arrange for a member of staff to monitor how quickly information about treatment and diagnosis is received about patients discharged from hospital. Establish if there is a significant risk arising from delays.

Stage 4: Make and carry out a learning and action plan

- Identify from six medical records the management plan for heart failure that you are following and compare this with the most recent guidelines. If there are gaps in your knowledge read up on the areas required. Discuss your findings with other members of the practice team.
- Study the results from the audit of the patients and their carers and decide what changes need to be made.
- Find out how other areas manage the transfer of information between hospitals and general practice on discharge. Make representations to your PCO to improve the communication between the hospitals you use and general practice.

Stage 5: Document your learning, competence, performance and standards of service delivery

- Record the results from your own review of your management of heart failure and the comments from other members of the practice team.

- Record the results of the audit and what changes are proposed. Plan to re-audit in 12 months.
- Record how other areas manage the transfer of information between hospitals and general practice on discharge. Record the results of your representations to your PCO to improve the communication between the hospitals you use and general practice.

Box 6.6:   Case study continued

Mrs Shelter re-attends with her daughter. The hospital has faxed you a copy of the discharge plan that had gone to her previous GP. You are able to make some minor changes to her regime, partly to simplify it and partly because of her most recent blood tests. You arrange for her to re-attend in two weeks when she and her daughter will have read through the patient information and can prepare a list of questions they want to discuss with you. You start to make a plan for her longer-term management.

Example cycle of evidence 6.3

- Focus: clinical care
- Other relevant foci: working with colleagues; relationships with patients; management

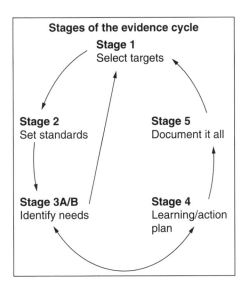

Stages of the evidence cycle

Stage 1 Select targets
Stage 2 Set standards
Stage 3A/B Identify needs
Stage 4 Learning/action plan
Stage 5 Document it all

Box 6.7:   Case study

Mr Waters' son rings to demand a visit. The receptionist tells you that the son had sounded quite angry on the phone. You refresh your memory about Mr Waters, who is 85 years of age, from his medical record. You are surprised to find that he has not been seen for five weeks, after having attended or had home visits for chronic heart failure quite frequently. You note that he has not had a recent repeat of his medication, but wonder if perhaps he has been staying with his son. You are rather alarmed to see that his last electrolyte results showed a low potassium level, and no action appears to have followed this. There is a handwritten note on the paper result that says: 'patient phoned and asked to attend', but no subsequent entry in the medical record. When you visit, Mr Waters is very poorly, his son furious with you and with him. Mr Waters says he does not want any more treatment, he has stopped his tablets and doesn't want any more blood tests.

> This is just an example. Keep your task simple. You could choose three or four cycles of evidence to demonstrate your competence each year.

Stage 1: Select your aspirations for good practice

The excellent GP:

- makes an adequate assessment of the patient's condition
- keeps comprehensive records outlining the management plan and information given to patients, including details of how results will be followed up and patients informed of results
- respects the autonomy of the patient to refuse examination, investigation and treatment
- arranges for appropriate supervision of staff and colleagues.

Stage 2: Set the standards for your outcomes

Outcomes might include:

- the way learning is applied
- a learnt skill
- a protocol
- a strategy that is implemented
- meeting recommended standards.

- Explore and record patients' decisions about examinations, investigation and treatment.
- Demonstrate consistent best practice in recalling patients after abnormal test results.

Stage 3A: Identify your learning needs

- Track your own actions when you receive abnormal results on ten occasions. Identify if you can take action if the patient does not attend for review.
- Use your reflective diary to record whether you are able to proactively discuss patients' feelings about continuing treatment and investigations in chronic illness.
- Reflect on how you manage the anger of relatives.

Stage 3B: Identify your service needs

Any of the needs assessment exercises in 3A may also reveal service needs.

- Track what happens to abnormal laboratory results when received by the practice.
- Discuss with practice staff if there is a way to identify when vulnerable patients do not attend, so that the relevant doctor or nurse can be informed and take action.
- Discuss with practice staff how they tell patients about their abnormal results and what feedback they can or should give to the responsible health professional.

Stage 4: Make and carry out a learning and action plan

- Compare your own actions on receiving abnormal test results with those commended by trusted colleagues or the local clinical tutor.
- Attend a workshop on identifying hidden depression in patients with chronic illnesses.
- Arrange a meeting with the practice staff to talk through how to manage the problem of vulnerable patients who do not attend when asked to do so.

Stage 5: Document your learning, competence, performance and standards of service delivery

- Record your observations about the changes you intend making to your practice as a result of attending the workshop. Plan to audit your management

of patients with chronic illness in 12 months to establish if you are any more likely to have discussed their feelings of helplessness and hopelessness.
- Record the changes made to the protocol for management of abnormal results referring to the key points you have learnt from colleagues.
- Record the suggestions from the reception staff about how to manage the non-attendance by vulnerable patients and how this had been implemented.

Box 6.8:   Case study continued

Mr Waters and his son calmed down when you expressed concern about his state of health and suggested that you all sat down to discuss how to manage the crisis. Mr Waters broke down in tears and his son said he would leave you to it, going out into the kitchen to make a cup of tea. You discussed the options and Mr Waters agreed to go into hospital for stabilisation.

When Mr Waters is discharged, he is on an antidepressant as well as all his other medication. Arrangements for home care have been put in place and the son has agreed to visit more regularly to help make his father feel that he has something to live for.

References

1   National Collaborating Centre for Chronic Conditions (2003) *Chronic Heart Failure: clinical guideline 5*. National Institute for Clinical Excellence, London. www.nice.org.uk.

2   Scottish Intercollegiate Guidelines Network (1999) *Diagnosis and Treatment of Heart Failure due to Left Ventricular Systolic Dysfunction*. SIGN, Edinburgh. www.sign.ac.uk.

3   NHS Executive (2000) *National Service Framework for Coronary Heart Disease*. Department of Health, London.

4   www.dh.gov.uk. Enter in the search box 'GPs with a special interest in echo-cardiography'.

5   Masoudi FA and Krumholz HM (2003) Polypharmacy and comorbidity in heart failure (Editorial). *British Medical Journal*. **327**: 513–14.

6   Swedberg K, Pfeffer M, Granger C *et al.* (1999) Candesartan in heart failure – assessment of reduction in mortality and morbidity (CHARM): rationale and design. Charm-Programme Investigators. *Journal of Cardiac Failure*. **5**: 276–82.

7   White H (2003) Candesartan and heart failure: the allure of CHARM (Editorial). *Lancet*. **362**: 754–5, and four fast-tracked papers, pages 759, 767, 772 and 777–8.

7

Cerebrovascular disease

Anterior circulation transient ischaemic attacks

Box 7.1: Case study

Mr Barrel, a 59-year-old publican who smokes 30 cigarettes a day, attends the evening surgery with an episode of loss of use in his right arm and leg lasting ten minutes.

What issues you should cover

Ask further questions about the nature of the neurological loss. Was it motor or sensory, was the face involved, were there any brainstem symptoms? (*See* Box 7.2 for likely symptoms.) Then ask questions about risk factors for arteriosclerosis. Questions about his modifiable risk factors, i.e. smoking, hypertension, hyperlipidaemia and diabetes, are particularly important.

Deal with the presenting condition

It is likely that Mr Barrel has had a transient ischaemic attack (TIA) in the territory of the left middle cerebral artery (*see* Box 7.2). He may have a tight stenosis of the left internal carotid artery that would be amenable to endarterectomy and reduce his risk of having a completed and disabling stroke. If Mr Barrel is a potential surgical candidate, he should have an urgent carotid ultrasound (Doppler).[1] This may be available via the local TIA or cerebrovascular clinic.

Box 7.2: Different presentations of problems with anterior and posterior cerebral circulation[2]

Anterior circulation

Hemiparesis (confined to one side of the body)

Hemisensory syndrome (face, arm and leg on one side of the body)

Dysphasia (affecting language, not articulation)

Visuospatial neglect (no knowledge of one side of the visual field and appearing to ignore visual and spatial cues coming from that direction)

Visual loss confined to one eye

Posterior circulation

Diplopia (seeing two images)

Vertigo (rotatory or tilting dizziness)

Nausea

Complete loss of vision or homonimous hemianopia (loss of corresponding halves of the one side of the field of vision in both eyes)

Crossed sensory syndrome[a]

Crossed motor syndrome[a]

([a] a defect involving one side of the face and the leg, trunk, or both on the other side)

If he had presented with diplopia and a weak arm then it would be likely that the TIA was in the posterior circulation (arising from a disturbance in blood supply in the vertebral–basilar system). Under those circumstances, a Doppler ultrasound of the carotid arteries would be inappropriate. Any stenosis identified would be asymptomatic. In general, in the UK, the risk from operating on asymptomatic carotid stenosis outweighs the potential advantage, though this is a matter of controversy.[3]

Whatever the Doppler results, it is important that Mr Barrel's modifiable risk factors for arteriosclerosis are minimised. Find out if he has hypertension. He should stop smoking and there are well-developed strategies for assisting in this process.[4] Although overall the success rate of interventions aimed to stop people smoking are disappointing, a TIA can have a profound psychological impact. Harness this fear in order to provide the motivation to become tobacco free.

Given the current epidemic of mature onset diabetes mellitus, all patients who have had a TIA should have a fasting glucose performed, unless they have been tested recently.

Fasting lipids provide both total cholesterol and LDL levels. The aim is to keep the total cholesterol below 5 mmol/l and the LDL below 3 mmol/l. As many people have already moved away from a traditional British diet of chips and bacon 'butties', diet alone rarely produces substantial falls in cholesterol levels. The statins are generally well tolerated and are very effective, both at lowering cholesterol and in reducing cerebrovascular and, more importantly in terms of numbers of people affected, cardiovascular mortality and morbidity.

Posterior circulation transient ischaemic attacks

> **Box 7.3:** Case study
>
> Mrs Fettler, a 68-year-old retired pottery worker, came to evening surgery complaining that earlier in the day the left side of her face, right arm and right leg had gone numb and been tingling for about 15 minutes. When she tried to walk, she was very unsteady. Now she felt completely back to normal apart from the fact she felt a bit washed out.

What issues you should cover

On enquiry, you find that Mrs Fettler does not have any of the usual modifiable risk factors for arteriosclerosis, but on examination, you discover that she has atrial fibrillation. The description of her event sounds like a posterior circulation TIA (*see* Box 7.2) and the most likely cause is an embolus arising from her heart. You need to establish if she has acute atrial fibrillation or if she is having episodes of paroxysmal atrial fibrillation. She is likely to have long-standing atrial fibrillation that has been previously undiagnosed. Look for the underlying risk factors for atrial fibrillation:

- ischaemic heart disease
- hypertension
- heart failure
- valve disease, especially following rheumatic heart disease
- diabetes
- alcohol abuse
- thyroid disease
- disorders of the lung or pleura.

You may need to obtain an opinion from a cardiologist to determine whether she is a candidate for cardioversion or rate-limiting medication. From the point of view of prevention of strokes, you will need to discuss with her the relative risks and benefits of aspirin versus warfarin for anti-embolic protection.[3]

Issues in the present consultation

In the absence of contraindications to full anticoagulation, the trial evidence would be in favour of full anticoagulation aiming for an international normalised ratio (INR) of 2 to 3.[1] However, some patients do not want to take 'rat poison'. They may have had a relative or friend die of the complications of warfarin, or the patient may just not like the idea. For others the notion of regular blood tests puts them off taking warfarin. The role of the medical adviser under these circumstances is to provide the patient with the information needed to make a decision and then support the patient in the decision they take. The evidence reported in the most recent Cochrane review suggests that anti-coagulant therapy can benefit people with non-rheumatic atrial fibrillation and recent cerebral ischaemia.[5] Aspirin may be a useful alternative if there is a contraindication to anticoagulant therapy. The risk of adverse events appears to be higher with anticoagulant therapy than aspirin. So, if Mrs Fettler is willing to have the regular blood checks necessary, the benefits of warfarin treatment probably outweigh the risks.

TIAs: implications for drivers

Box 7.4:   Case study

Mr Driver attends surgery after an episode of altered sensation in his left hand and intense rotational vertigo. This is the third time it has happened. He had ignored the previous episodes, but this time he was driving his lorry through road works on the motorway and knocked over a few cones before he got the lorry back under control.

What issues you should cover

Further details of the attacks should be elicited if they are available. These sound like posterior circulation TIAs (*see* Box 7.2), but additional evidence such as complaints of nausea or diplopia would be useful. Ask Mr Driver if he had made any sudden neck movements that may have compromised the blood flow in a vertebral artery in the neck and provoked the attack.

Evaluate Mr Driver's risk factors for arteriosclerosis and start him on an antiplatelet regimen unless he has contraindications, such as a previous history of a peptic ulcer.

Issues in the present consultation

The reason that Mr Driver came to the surgery was that he nearly had a crash. It is clearly unsafe for him to continue to drive for the present. The Driver and Vehicle Licensing Agency (DVLA) takes the following position with regard to vocational driving licences:

> Recommend refusal/revocation for at least 12 months following a stroke or TIA. Can be considered for licensing after this period if there is a full and complete recovery and there are no other significant risk factors. Licensing will also be subject to satisfactory medical reports including exercise ECG testing.[6]

Most vocational licence holders understand the stringent rules with regard to health and it will come as no surprise to Mr Driver that he will not be able to drive his lorry, or a car, for a while. However, you will need to talk through with him the problems of not being able to work in his usual occupation for at least 12 months.

The regulations for ordinary driving licence holders who have a cerebrovascular event are less stringent:

> Must not drive for at least 1 month.
> May resume driving after this time if the clinical recovery is satisfactory.
> There is no need to notify DVLA *unless* there is residual neurological deficit at 1 month, particularly:
> * visual field defects
> * cognitive defects
> * impaired limb function.
> Minor limb weakness alone will not require notification unless restriction to certain types of vehicle or vehicles with adapted controls is needed. Adaptations may be able to overcome severe physical impairment.[6]

TIA symptoms in oral contraceptive users

Box 7.5: Case study

Miss Alarm is a 16-year-old woman who has been on the combined oral contraceptive pill for three months. The pill is suiting her well, but she has had an episode of weakness in her left leg and hand lasting half an hour. This has fully resolved.

What issues you should cover

Further details of the neurological event are needed. In particular, look for evidence of another diagnosis such as migraine. The development of a unilateral headache with photophobia, phonophobia and nausea about half an hour to an hour after the episode of weakness would be suggestive of migraine.

You should specifically ask about any history of recent trauma to the neck, such as a whiplash from a road traffic accident or a family history of thromboembolic events.

Issues in the present consultation

If an alternative diagnosis is not apparent, then you will have to presume she may have had a TIA. Causes of TIA and cerebral infarction other than arteriosclerosis are listed in Box 7.6. If you have made a diagnosis of focal migraine, or if you think she may have had a TIA, then combined oral contraceptives containing oestrogen are contraindicated because of their prothrombotic effects. She should stop the combined oral contraceptive and use an alternative form of contraception. She could use a progestogen-only pill, injection or implant or a non-hormonal method such as a barrier method with the backup of emergency contraception. She could have an intrauterine device fitted, although this might not be the first choice for a nulliparous woman. She should start on 75 mg of aspirin a day and be referred for investigation by a consultant neurologist.

Box 7.6:   Causes of TIA and cerebral infarction other than atherosclerosis (these causes are more common in younger people)

- Combined oral contraceptive pill
- Cardioembolic causes
  - patent foramen ovale
  - valvular disease
- Arrhythmia
- Dissection of carotid or vertebral arteries
- Prothrombotic tendencies
  - protein S and C deficiencies
  - antithrombin III deficiency
  - lupus anticoagulant syndrome
- Vasculitis
- Complex migraine

Surgical options for treatment

Box 7.7:   Case study

Mrs Nelson is an 80-year-old widow who had a minor myocardial infarct three years ago and has been on aspirin, atenolol and a low fat diet since. She presents with an episode of loss of vision in the left eye. This lasted five minutes and then fully resolved. Two weeks previously she had had an episode lasting 15 minutes of loss of use of her right hand with some difficulty getting her words out, which she had ignored. Examination reveals a harsh bruit over the bifurcation in her left carotid artery.

What issues you should cover

Ask specific questions about any previous episodes of neurological dysfunction and check her adherence to her current drug regimen. It is likely that Mrs Nelson is having TIAs arising from a stenosis at the bifurcation of the left carotid artery.

Issues in the present consultation

Mrs Nelson requires urgent carotid Doppler measurement to determine if the stenosis is 70% or greater. If it is, then an urgent vascular surgical opinion is necessary with a surgeon who frequently undertakes carotid endarterectomy. Ideally, find out the surgeon's audited complication rate, as the balance between the probabilities of benefit and harm under these circumstances depends on the risks of surgery.[3] Auscultation is a very poor method of excluding a tight stenosis. All patients who have had a TIA or minor cerebral infarction and who are potential candidates for surgery should have a Doppler ultrasound. However, if a harsh bruit is heard on the appropriate side, this increases the probability that a potentially surgically remediable stenosis will be present.

Her modifiable risk factors for arteriosclerosis appear to be hypertension and hyperlipidaemia. She is a non-smoker, but a fasting glucose level will be required, as she could have developed mature onset diabetes mellitus. In addition, her fasting lipids will need reassessing. There has been some controversy over the use of statins in people over 70 years old, but the consensus view is that provided an older person's life expectancy is greater than two years, it is appropriate to use statins, if diet alone is ineffective in reducing total cholesterol to acceptable levels.[7]

Despite being on aspirin, Mrs Nelson is at significant risk of going on to have a disabling stroke. Some practitioners would add in a second antiplatelet drug. There is controversy over whether to use aspirin and dipyridamole, or aspirin and clopidogrel. The latter regimen is probably more effective, but currently we do not know if there is a price to pay in terms of increased rate of intracerebral haemorrhage for that greater efficacy.[8] There are more clinical trials in progress that should answer this question.

Stroke management

Box 7.8:   Case study

The receptionist puts a call through from Mr Convoy's wife on your way to the morning surgery. Mrs Convoy tells you that when she took her husband, a 58-year-old coach driver, a cup of tea in bed this morning, his face had sagged and he couldn't talk to her properly. He had tried to get out of bed and fallen over. He had been late home the previous night and had seemed fine then. She is distraught and wants you to come straight away. You divert to their house and confirm your impression that Mr Convoy has had a stroke. On direct questioning, he has had no vomiting, dizziness or headache. You give him 300 mg of aspirin and arrange to admit him immediately. You ask for an urgent ambulance.

Management of transient ischaemic attacks and stroke

The National Service Framework (NSF) for Older People for England sets out actions in relation to the care of patients with stroke.[8] This process is subject to a timetable (*see* Box 7.9).

Box 7.9:   National Service Framework for Older People for England[8]

April 2002: every hospital caring for stroke patients will have plans to introduce a stroke service in accordance with the stroke service model in the NSF.
April 2003: every hospital will establish clinical audit systems based on the Royal College of Physicians' guidelines for the management of stroke.[1]
April 2004: PCTs will ensure that –

- all practices use protocols agreed with local experts to treat and identify patients at risk of stroke
- all GP practices have an agreed protocol for rapid referral for TIA
- all GP practices can identify patients who have had a stroke and are caring for them according to agreed protocols
- every general practice has established clinical audit systems for stroke.

One hundred per cent of all hospitals looking after patients who have had a stroke will have a specialised service as described in the stroke service model.

Quality indicators in stroke and transient ischaemic attacks

The quality points available under the new GP contract are achievable on a sliding scale, so while you are collecting the data to demonstrate your own competence you are also helping to show that your practice is achieving high standards of care. Quality points in this domain are very similar to those for coronary heart disease:

- a register of patients with stroke or transient ischaemic attacks: 4 points
- 80% of patients with a presumptive diagnosis of stroke have been referred for confirmation of the diagnosis by CT or MRI scan: 2 points
- 90% of patients on the register have their smoking status recorded: 3 points
- 70% of patients on the register who smoke have been offered smoking cessation advice in the last 15 months: 2 points
- 90% of patients on the register have a record of their blood pressure in the last 15 months: 2 points
- 70% of patients on the stroke register have a blood pressure on treatment of less than that recommended by the British Hypertension Society Guidelines:[9] 5 points
- 90% of patients on the stroke register have their cholesterol level recorded in the last 15 months: 2 points
- 60% of patients on the stroke register have a cholesterol level on treatment of 5 mmol/l or less in the last 15 months: 5 points
- 90% of patients on the stroke register with a non-haemorrhagic event are on antithrombotic therapy: 4 points
- 85% of patients on the stroke register have received the influenza immunisation in the previous September to March: 2 points.

Exception reporting will be the same as for coronary heart disease (*see* page 71), so make sure that you record your discussions.

The recommendations for optimal management of TIA and stroke overleaf are taken from the TIA and Stroke Clinic at the University Hospital of North Staffordshire (*see* Box 7.10).[10]

Box 7.10: Current advice from the North Staffordshire cerebrovascular (TIA) clinic[10]

Antiplatelet agents in use:
- aspirin 75–150 mg daily
- dipyridamole modified release 200 mg twice daily
- clopidogrel 75 mg daily

Use of antiplatelet agents:
- first-line or low risk: aspirin alone
- high risk and failed control with aspirin: combined aspirin and dipyridamole
- alternatives to aspirin: dipyridamole or clopidogrel

They are based on:

- the Royal College of Physicians' guidelines for the management of stroke 2002.[1] A full version is also available on the Internet[1]
- the National Service Framework for Coronary Heart Disease (and other occlusive vascular disease).[11]

Acute treatment

- Aspirin (300 mg) should be given as soon as possible after the onset of stroke symptoms (if a diagnosis of haemorrhage is considered unlikely).
- No other drug treatment aimed at treatment of the stroke should be given unless as part of a randomised controlled trial.
- Where stroke has caused weak or paralysed legs, full-length compression stockings should be applied (unless contraindicated) to prevent venous thrombosis.

Secondary prevention

- All patients should have their blood pressure checked, and hypertension persisting for over one month should be treated. Follow the British Hypertension Society guidelines for optimal blood pressure treatment.[9]
- All patients not on anticoagulation should be taking aspirin 75 mg daily, or a combination of low-dose aspirin and dipyridamole modified release (MR). Where patients are aspirin intolerant, an alternative antiplatelet agent (clopidogrel 75 mg daily or dipyridamole MR 200 mg twice daily) should be used.

- In the presence of atrial fibrillation, mitral valve disease, prosthetic heart valves, or within three months of myocardial infarction, anticoagulation should be considered for all patients who have had an ischaemic stroke. (Anticoagulation after transient ischaemic attacks or minor strokes is contraindicated unless cardiac embolism is suspected.)
- Any patient with a carotid artery area stroke, and minor or absent residual disability should be considered for carotid Doppler scanning with a view to endarterectomy if a surgically significant stenosis is detected.
- All smokers should receive advice about how to stop smoking including advice on the use of nicotine replacement therapy.
- All patients should be given advice on physical activity, diet, weight and alcohol consumption.
- Statins and dietary advice should be given to all patients to either lower total cholesterol to less than 5 mmol/l (LDL-C to less than 3 mmol/l) or by 30% (whichever is the greater).
- Meticulous control of hypertension (130/80 mmHg or lower) should be used and glycaemic control in those with diabetes (haemoglobin A1c (HbA1c) 7.0% or lower).

Management of the acute episode and its aftercare

It is recommended that patients who develop a stroke should be admitted to hospital and be cared for in a designated stroke unit. Thrombolysis within three hours of a stroke is now a licensed treatment, so rapid admission should be the rule, just as for a suspected heart attack. It has been suggested that the name 'stroke' should be changed to 'brain attack' to galvanise people into rapid action. Multidisciplinary staff in a stroke unit can provide rehabilitation based on specialised assessment. Recovery is quicker and complications are avoided by staff adopting the correct approach.[12] In 2003, only 36% of patients admitted with a stroke spend any time on a stroke unit, although 75% of hospitals now have a stroke unit.

The NSF for Older People recommends that all patients with an acute stroke should have a CT scan within 48 hours to help to decide on whether they should take antiplatelet medication.[8]

Care pathways – a flow diagram of how a patient will have his or her care delivered and managed – should be created for the long-term care of stroke patients and their carers and should not finish on discharge (the current situation for many patients). This care pathway must be relevant to local circumstances. It needs to include all the people and services relevant to the care of the patient. For example, practice nurses can be key in providing primary and secondary prevention care, and physiotherapists can sometimes organise exercise on prescription at local gyms. Counsellors can offer support for longer-term emotional issues and depression should be treated. Speech therapy, although in short supply, can be very helpful for dysphasia and some speech therapists have special skills in diagnosing swallowing difficulties.

Before Mr Convoy is discharged, alternative environments for ongoing care need to be considered. Assessment and ongoing rehabilitation are often better provided in settings other than hospitals e.g. own home, housing-based intermediate care, care homes and community hospitals, with nurse/therapy-led services. If a stroke has altered someone's level of independence significantly they need time and a different environment, other than acute care, to decide what is best for them and their carers. Particular difficulties may arise because of patients' disabilities, dysphasia, dysphagia and with depression.

Patients and their relatives need reliable information about what has happened, what they might expect during recovery and how they can help themselves. Encourage them to contact the Stroke Association which has a whole range of booklets and leaflets written in everyday language.[13] As well as supplying written information, the staff at regional centres will try to answer specific questions, or refer patients or relatives to other organisations that can help. The community service, Family Support, is a visiting service that provides emotional support in the early days after the stroke and over the time when the patient goes home. This is an expanding service not available in all areas. If there is one in your area the stroke care co-ordinator will lend a sympathetic ear to problems, suggest practical solutions, and point patients and relatives towards all the help they are entitled to. The Stroke Association also helps to run stroke clubs of which there are more than 40 throughout the UK. Some of these offer therapy and others are just social.

Collecting data to demonstrate your learning, competence, performance and standards of service delivery

Example cycle of evidence 7.1

- Focus: clinical care
- Other relevant foci: relationships with patients; working with colleagues

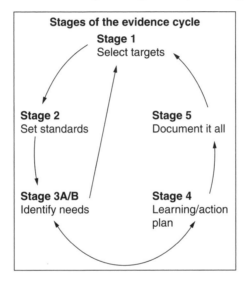

Stages of the evidence cycle

Stage 1
Select targets

Stage 2
Set standards

Stage 5
Document it all

Stage 3A/B
Identify needs

Stage 4
Learning/action plan

Box 7.11: Case study

Mr Ladder, a 70-year-old retired painter and decorator, presents with a 'funny turn'. He was up a stepladder cleaning a gutter when he suddenly felt light-headed. He lost his vision and felt that he was about to fall. When his vision returned he could see two television aerials on top of his bungalow and his left hand could not grip as strongly as the right. He gently came down the ladder and lay on the lawn until his wife found him half an hour later. By then, he was beginning to feel better, but it was not until the next day that he was back to normal.

This is just an example. Keep your task simple. You could choose three or four cycles of evidence to demonstrate your competence each year.

Stage 1: Select your aspirations for good practice

The excellent GP:

- has the knowledge and skills to recognise the symptoms suggestive of posterior versus anterior cerebral circulation disturbance
- knows how to explain the management of TIAs to patients to promote concordance with therapy.

Stage 2: Set the standards for your outcomes

Outcomes might include:

- the way learning is applied
- a learnt skill
- a protocol
- a strategy that is implemented
- meeting recommended standards.

- Primary care team members know the difference between symptoms and signs of posterior and anterior circulatory disturbance.
- Carotid Doppler studies are not requested for patients with posterior circulatory disturbances.
- Explanations to patients about their TIA are based on up-to-date guidelines.

Stage 3A: Identify your learning needs

- Self-assess your knowledge of cerebral vasculature. Self-assess your knowledge of symptoms arising from posterior circulatory disturbance.
- Carry out a significant event audit of a patient who has had a stroke following a TIA.

Stage 3B: Identify your service needs

Any of the needs assessment exercises in 3A may also reveal service needs.

- Review the pathways whereby the practice obtains carotid Doppler ultrasounds.
- Audit the last five Doppler ultrasounds undertaken and identify if they were requested appropriately.

- Check the availability of guidelines about the management of TIAs and if they are up to date.

Stage 4: Make and carry out a learning and action plan

- Read up about the blood supply of the brain.
- Read about the likely symptoms arising from dysfunction of various parts of the brain.
- Review the patient information leaflets about stroke to assess if they are up to date with current guidelines.
- Find out how patients are managed by the local TIA or neurological referral clinic by attending a talk by the consultant or sitting in on the clinic.

Stage 5: Document your learning, competence, performance and standards of service delivery

- Make a record of testing yourself (pencil and paper) by drawing the circle of Willis.
- List the symptoms and signs most likely to be associated with anterior and posterior circulatory disorders.
- Keep the audit results of the appropriateness of the carotid Doppler requests.
- Write a description of the significant event audit and the subsequent action taken.
- Keep a copy of the up-to-date guidelines for the management of TIAs and the record of its availability to clinical staff.

Box 7.12:   Case study continued

Mr Ladder is found to have diabetes and an associated hypertriglyceridaemia. His TIA was in the posterior circulation, so no Doppler ultrasound was required. His diabetes is controlled through diet. Regular exercise and weight loss reduce his blood pressure. He is started on aspirin 75 mg a day and dipyridamole 200 mg MR twice a day. At his medication review appointment a year later, he has had no further episodes.

Example cycle of evidence 7.2

- Focus: clinical care
- Other relevant focus: relationships with patients

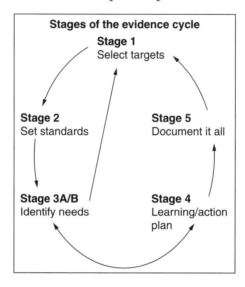

Box 7.13:   Case study

Mr Gear is a 68-year-old retired fitter who has come to see you after spending a week in hospital. The discharge slip diagnosis is 'stroke' and Mr Gear tells you his right side went weak, but has largely recovered. He smokes 20 cigarettes a day, is obese and has a blood pressure of 190/90 mmHg. A year ago, he had a fasting total cholesterol of 6 mmol/l and a fasting glucose of 7.2 mmol/l.

This is just an example. Keep your task simple. You could choose three or four cycles of evidence to demonstrate your competence each year.

Stage 1: Select your aspirations for good practice

The excellent GP:

- is always on the lookout for modifiable risk factors for arteriosclerosis.

Stage 2: Set the standards for your outcomes

Outcomes might include:
- the way learning is applied
- a learnt skill
- a protocol
- a strategy that is implemented
- meeting recommended standards.

- Every patient attending the surgery with a cerebrovascular event has a review of their risk factors for arteriosclerosis in a similar way to best practice for those who have had cardiovascular events.[9]

Stage 3A: Identify your learning needs

- Self-assess your knowledge for the targets for blood pressure, lipids and diabetic control in people who have had a TIA.
- Use your reflective diary to record how you communicate the risks discovered to patients.

Stage 3B: Identify your service needs

Any of the needs assessment exercises in 3A may also reveal service needs.

- Review the notes of the last ten patients in whom a diagnosis of stroke or TIA was made six to twelve months previously. Record if their risk factors were identified and managed before and/or after the event.
- Review the practice protocols for stroke and coronary artery disease to ensure that patients with cerebrovascular disease have their risk factors managed in a similar way to best practice for those with coronary artery disease.[9]

Stage 4: Make and carry out a learning and action plan

- Run an in-house training event surrounding risk factor management in cerebrovascular disease.
- Put the agreed guidelines on management of risk factors in cerebrovascular disease into the practice computer system so that they are available to all partners during a consultation.

Stage 5: Document your learning, competence, performance and standards of service delivery

- Record your management of ten consecutive patients who present with cerebrovascular disease.
- Keep a reflective diary for a week on how often you are able to identify and communicate to patients their modifiable risk factors for arteriosclerosis before events.
- Repeat the review of the notes of the next ten patients in whom a diagnosis of stroke or TIA is made, as to whether their risk factors have been identified and managed after the learning event.
- Keep a copy of the practice protocols for stroke and coronary artery disease.

Box 7.14:   Case study continued

Mr Gear has a 'full house' of the modifiable risk factors for arteriosclerosis. He goes onto the smoking cessation programme with nicotine replacement. He starts a diet and fasting lipids and glucose are arranged. You ask him to have his blood pressure checked by the practice nurse on two occasions to determine if his hypertension is sustained, and arrange to see him again to start therapy if indicated. He has promised to start a gentle exercise programme.

Example cycle of evidence 7.3

- Focus: teaching and training
- Other relevant foci: relationships with patients; maintaining good medical practice; probity

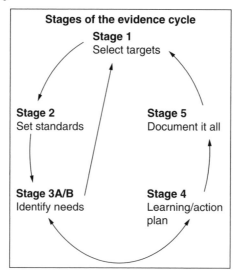

Stages of the evidence cycle

Stage 1
Select targets

Stage 2
Set standards

Stage 5
Document it all

Stage 3A/B
Identify needs

Stage 4
Learning/action plan

Box 7.15: Case study

A medical student is shadowing you to gain experience about working in general practice. Mrs Shepherd is a 70-year-old widowed farmer's wife who lives in an isolated farmhouse. She calls you out to see her after she has had an episode of facial weakness with slurring of speech lasting half an hour. Her only modifiable risk factor appears to be her hypertension. She is already taking bendrofluazide. You consider adding an ACE inhibitor, but decide to monitor her blood pressure for a while. You start her on an aspirin 75 mg a day. You tell her that she will not be able to drive for at least a month, but can restart if she has no more episodes. The medical student comments on the way back that he thinks you should not have told Mrs Shepherd about the driving restrictions as she will lose her independence. The student comments that in this isolated area surely it would not make any difference if Mrs Shepherd drove her car occasionally.

> This is just an example. Keep your task simple. You could choose three or four cycles of evidence to demonstrate your competence each year.

Stage 1: Select your aspirations for good practice

The excellent GP:

- has a working knowledge of the DVLA rules with regard to driving and knows where to look to check
- can help patients to comply with the law and look for ways to mitigate the effects
- is able to explain the rationale behind the decision to act within the law.

Stage 2: Set the standards for your outcomes

Outcomes might include:

- the way learning is applied
- a learnt skill
- a protocol
- a strategy that is implemented
- meeting recommended standards.

- The advice about the driving regulations given to patients who have had a cardiovascular event is recorded in their medical records.
- You can communicate the reasons for abiding by the driving licence regulations and show how to mitigate the effects.

Stage 3A: Identify your learning needs

- Self-assess knowledge of the driving regulations. Identify where you would look to get up-to-date information.[6]

Stage 3B: Identify your service needs

Any of the needs assessment exercises in 3A may also reveal service needs.

- Informally ask colleagues if they are aware of the driving licence regulations.
- Review the electronic system in practice to identify if such information is easily accessible.
- Check whether the syllabus for the medical student includes ethical and probity issues.
- Ask the practice manager to establish what local help is available for isolated patients without their own transport.

Stage 4: Make and carry out a learning and action plan

- Run an in-house training event, that the medical student can attend, around driving regulations and patients who have had strokes.
- Arrange for the driving licence regulations to be easily accessible via the electronic system in your practice.

Stage 5: Document your learning, competence, performance and standards of service delivery

- Evaluate your training session by recording the opinions of colleagues about whether it met their needs and they were more confident of the regulations.
- Record your discussion with the medical student about the ethical and probity implications of advising patients about the driving regulations.
- Keep a copy of the information about the driving licence regulations that is given routinely to patients you see following a cerebrovascular event.

- Ensure that a copy of the local resources for isolated patients without their own transport is added to the practice leaflet.

Box 7.16: Case study continued

Mrs Shepherd is very upset when you tell her that she cannot drive her car for a month as this leaves her very isolated. You encourage her to contact her son who lives locally. He takes her shopping and on other trips into the village. She comments at the end of the month that this has been the most she has seen of him for the last few years. She also uses the community bus that takes people to the weekly local market and meets several old friends. She has no more cerebrovascular events and resumes driving, but continues to see more of her son. You let the medical student know the outcome for this patient.

Example cycle of evidence 7.4

- Focus: keeping up to date
- Other relevant focus: relationships with patients

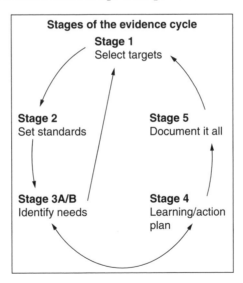

Box 7.17: Case study

Mr Flow is a 47-year-old businessman who is a heavy smoker, but is otherwise healthy. He has an episode of loss of vision in his left eye. A carotid Doppler test demonstrates a 30% stenosis of the left internal carotid above the bifurcation. He has no other identifiable risk factors for arteriosclerosis.

> This is just an example. Keep your task simple. You could choose three or four cycles of evidence to demonstrate your competence each year.

Stage 1: Select your aspirations for good practice

The excellent GP:

- is aware of the antiplatelet drugs available, their side-effect profile, efficacy and cost.

Stage 2: Set the standards for your outcomes

Outcomes might include:

- the way learning is applied
- a learnt skill
- a protocol
- a strategy that is implemented
- meeting recommended standards.

- Every patient who is at increased risk of atherosclerotic events takes an antiplatelet agent unless contraindicated.
- Update or compose a practice protocol for prescribing antiplatelet agents.

Stage 3A: Identify your learning needs

- Self-assess your knowledge of the available antiplatelet agents and the trial evidence supporting their use.
- List the common side-effects associated with each of the three agents: aspirin, dipyridamole and clopidogrel.[14]

Stage 3B: Identify your service needs

Any of the needs assessment exercises in 3A may also reveal service needs.

- Informally ask GP colleagues what their policy is with regard to the use of antiplatelet agents.

- Determine if the practice has an up-to-date guideline for the use of these drugs that is in line with current recommendations.

Stage 4: Make and carry out a learning and action plan

- Run an in-house training event providing the evidence to support the use of the various antiplatelet agents, their side-effects and relative costs.
- Make or update the practice prescribing guideline.

Stage 5: Document your learning, competence, performance and standards of service delivery

- Record the practice consensus for the guidelines for the use of these drugs.
- Carry out an audit of comparing the prescription of dipyridamole and clopidogrel in ten patients with the agreed practice guidelines.

Box 7.18:   Case study continued

You start Mr Flow on 75 mg aspirin a day, but he has a further TIA two weeks later. You add in dipyridamole MR 200 mg twice a day. Unfortunately, he develops continuing diarrhoea, which causes him to stop the dipyridamole, so you add in 75 mg of clopidogrel instead.

Example cycle of evidence 7.5

- Focus: good medical practice
- Other relevant foci: relationships with patients; working with colleagues

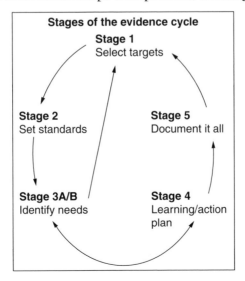

Stages of the evidence cycle

Box 7.19:   Case study

Mrs Dipper is a 77-year-old retired pottery worker who presents with a right hemiparesis involving her face, arm and leg, which resolved over two days. She has a harsh bruit over the bifurcation of her left carotid artery. She had a myocardial infarction ten years previously, but is otherwise well. You make a referral to your local TIA clinic, but are dismayed to discover the waiting time is three months.

> This is just an example. Keep your task simple. You could choose three or four cycles of evidence to demonstrate your competence each year.

Stage 1: Select your aspirations for good practice

The excellent GP:

- is aware of the referral routes available to get appropriate care for his/her patient.

Stage 2: Set the standards for your outcomes

Outcomes might include:

- the way learning is applied
- a learnt skill
- a protocol
- a strategy that is implemented
- meeting recommended standards.

- The GP practice has an agreed protocol for rapid referral for TIAs.
- Alternative referral strategies are considered when the usual route is inappropriately slow.

Stage 3A: Identify your learning needs

- Review what alternative referral routes for rapid referral for TIA assessment are known to you and the likely waiting times.

- Look for information on best practice for referral for TIAs, e.g. on the National electronic Library for Health.[15]

Stage 3B: Identify your service needs

> Any of the needs assessment exercises in 3A may also reveal service needs.

- Informally ask GP colleagues which referral route they would use under similar circumstances.
- Ask the relevant director in the local PCO, who is responsible for commissioning services, what arrangements have been made for rapid referral of patients with TIA.

Stage 4: Make and carry out a learning and action plan

- Find out the waiting times for TIA clinics/vascular clinics in neighbouring hospital(s).
- Identify if direct access for carotid Doppler is available.
- Discuss with the PCO about arranging an appropriately rapid referral route for your patients.

Stage 5: Document your learning, competence, performance and standards of service delivery

- Record information if GP colleagues have identified faster ways of getting your patient the appropriate test.
- Record the correspondence, including your evidence about best practice, with the chief executive of the PCO as to what the procedure is to get appropriately rapid referrals.

Box 7.20:   Case study continued

You telephone the consultant in charge of the TIA clinic who arranges an urgent carotid Doppler for Mrs Dipper without her being seen in the clinic. This demonstrates an 80% stenosis of the left internal carotid. The patient is fast tracked into the clinic and after appropriate counselling and further investigations she is referred for a carotid endarterectomy.

References

1   The Intercollegiate Working Party for Stroke (2002) *National Clinical Guidelines for Stroke*. Royal College of Physicians, London. Also available on www.eguidelines.co.uk, full version at www.rcplondon.ac.uk/pubs/books/stroke/index.htm.

2   Ellis SJ (1997) *Clinical Neurology: essential concepts.* Butterworth-Heinemann, Oxford.

3   Godlee F (ed.) (2003) *Clinical Evidence Concise.* BMJ Publishing Group, London. www.clinicalevidence.com.

4   Centre for Reviews and Dissemination (1998) Smoking cessation: what the health service can do. *Effectiveness Matters* Vol. 3 Issue 1. Also available from http://www.york.ac.uk/inst/crd/crdpublications.htm.

5   Koudstaal PJ (2003) Anticoagulants versus antiplatelet therapy for preventing stroke in patients with nonrheumatic atrial fibrillation and a history of stroke or transient ischemic attacks (Cochrane Review). *The Cochrane Library, Issue 4, 2002.* Update Software, Oxford.

6   Department for Transport (version August 2003 updated every six months) *UK Driving Licence Regulations for Neurological Conditions.* www.dvla.gov.uk/at_a_glance/ch1_neurological.htm.

7   Barnett HJM, Eliasziw M and Meldrum HE (1999) Prevention of ischaemic stroke. *British Medical Journal.* **318**: 1539–43.

8   Philp I and Platt D (2001) *National Service Framework for Older People.* Department of Health, London.

9   Foord-Kelcey G (ed.) (2003) *Guidelines* vol. 20. Medendium Group Publishing Ltd, Berkhamsted. www.eguidelines.co.uk.

10 Welton M, Ellis SJ and Lunn F (2002) *Optimal Management of TIA and Stroke.* Cerebrovascular (TIA) Clinic, North Staffordshire Hospital, University Hospital of North Staffordshire, Stoke-on-Trent.

11 www.dh.gov.uk/assetRoot/04/04/90/70/04049070.pdf.

12 The Service Improvement Team, NHS Modernisation Agency (2002) *National Service Framework for Older People November – what makes a good stroke service and how do we get there?* Department of Health, London. www.dh.gov.uk/assetRoot/04/01/95/54/04019554.pdf.

13 www.stroke.org.uk. Tel: +44 (0)845 30 33 100 for details of local contacts.

14 Joint Formulary Committee (2003) *British National Formulary.* British Medical Association and Royal Pharmaceutical Society, London. www.bnf.org.

15 www.nelh.nhs.uk.

8

Headache

Complaints of headache account for as many as a quarter of new patients referred to neurologists.

Tension headaches

Box 8.1:   Case study

Miss Tension plonked herself down and described her headaches, rubbing her forehead with her right hand as she spoke. The pressing ache felt like a tight band around her head that could last for a few hours to whole days. The headaches had been present for years off and on, but had become a daily occurrence since her partner had left her as she struggled to combine a full-time job with looking after her young son. She was still able to go about her normal activities when the headaches were in full fling – they did not stop her from doing her job or domestic tasks at home.

What issues you should cover

Headache is a common symptom that rarely has a serious cause. Miss Tension's symptoms fit with a diagnosis of tension headache, being bilateral and not prohibiting her from going about her everyday activities.[1,2] The definition of chronic tension-type headache is one showing the following features:

- headaches on 15 or more days per month for at least six months
- pain that is bilateral, pressing, or tightening in quality
- pain of mild or moderate intensity
- activities not prevented by the headache
- pain not aggravated by routine physical activity
- the presence of no more than one additional clinical feature of nausea, photophobia or phonophobia
- no vomiting.[3]

Many people with chronic tension-type headaches do not consult a doctor about them. As many as one in 25 of the population are thought to suffer from daily or near-daily headaches.[2,4] Tension-type headaches are more common in women. Nearly half of people suffering from chronic tension-type headaches have a family history of such headaches.

During the description of the headache symptoms, you will be ruling out any serious underlying cause. Check that any neurological symptoms disappear between attacks when your patient is pain free. In the history you will be looking out for other symptoms such as:

- acute onset (e.g. onset measured in seconds suggests an intracranial haemorrhage, which is often described as 'like a blow to the head', more gradual but acute onset might suggest infection, benign intracranial hypertension, or a space-occupying lesion)
- worsening with exertion (e.g. migraine, raised intracranial pressure)
- rash (e.g. meningitis, or the headache accompanying a pyrexial illness)
- indications of a neurological deficit (e.g. an intracranial tumour, abscess or haematoma)
- behavioural change (e.g. often reported by friends or relatives and suggestive of raised intracranial pressure)
- vomiting (e.g. migraine, benign intracranial hypertension, meningitis)
- head injury (e.g. haematoma or haemorrhage).

Examination will include recording a blood pressure reading (hypertension is rarely a cause of headache, but measuring blood pressure is expected by patients and useful for your quality points). Any neurological symptoms will prompt a search for neurological signs. You could examine the fundi to look for papilloedema due to benign intracranial hypertension. Although, if you are not confident that you can exclude papilloedema by fundoscopy and your index of suspicion is high, you would organise investigations anyway.

Chat to Miss Tension about reducing the pressures of her lifestyle. Advise her about taking simple analgesics or NSAIDs. Warn Miss Tension to avoid over-use of analgesics and to limit the amount she takes for her headaches. One review of the research indicated that taking common analgesics several times per week, over considerable time, may cause rather than relieve headaches.[2] Find out what medication she has been buying over the counter. Caffeine- and codeine-containing analgesics can trigger medication-overuse headaches. A good rule of thumb is not to use analgesics for more than seven days a month. If additional pain relief is needed, then aspirin is not thought to cause daily analgesic headaches.

Some doctors recommend amitriptyline starting at 10 mg at night and slowly increasing the dose until the headaches are contained. There is some research that has found that amitriptyline reduces the duration and frequency of moderate to severe chronic tension-type headaches, but the benefits may not be outweighed by the risks of dependence.[2]

Some non-pharmacological treatments may help. There is inconclusive research that acupuncture, cognitive behaviour therapy and relaxation therapy may help chronic tension headaches.[2]

Intracranial tumours

Box 8.2:   Case study

Mr Aspen is brought to see you by his daughter because he had what appeared to be a fit the day before, while he was visiting his daughter's home. He had lost consciousness without warning and had a generalised convulsion, then been a bit drowsy afterwards. His daughter had wanted to call out the emergency doctor but Mr Aspen had refused as he had several similar 'funny dos' in the last few weeks. He had also noticed pins and needles lasting for a few minutes, from time to time, in his right arm leaving it weak afterwards. Mr Aspen had come to see one of your GP colleagues several months ago complaining of newly occurring headaches and had already been referred to a neurologist, but was still waiting to be seen.

What issues you should cover

You will know that brain tumours commonly present with focal seizures, behaviour change and/or neurological deficits and that new onset headache may be a feature, as for Mr Aspen. Two in five intracranial tumours are metastatic, many of which are of bronchial origin. So, you can look through Mr Aspen's history and note whether he is known to have had a primary cancer and what his smoking habits have been.

You will want to do a brief survey of his cranial nerves and neurological system for any impairments and look at his general state of health and ability to function independently.

You will know that it is likely that Mr Aspen does have a space-occupying lesion and will refer him to a neurologist under the two week cancer-referral system unless you feel his clinical state warrants an emergency admission. You may be able to arrange a MRI scan, although this is not available as a primary care referral in some areas.

Temporal arteritis

Box 8.3:   Case study

Mrs Coot is a 75-year-old lady who has come to see you for two reasons – because she feels so worn out and because of her headaches. Amongst the many symptoms she describes in minute detail, you pick out that she mentions that her scalp is so tender it is stopping her from wearing a hat as she usually does.

What issues you should cover

Giant cell or temporal arteritis affects elderly people and mainly women. The arteritis can involve inflammation of the lining of almost any large artery – carotid, vertebral, meningeal and, more rarely, intracerebral arteries. About half of those with giant cell arteritis have symptoms of polymyalgia rheumatica (PMR). In temporal arteritis, the scalp is usually exquisitely tender to touch. Patients may complain that they cannot brush their hair or put their head on the pillow at night.

Headache in temporal arteritis is usually accompanied by systemic symptoms. Ask Mrs Coot if she has experienced weight loss and night sweats as well as the lassitude she has described – all common symptoms of temporal arteritis. Other symptoms to enquire about might include arthralgia, anorexia, low-grade fever and depression.

You will need to confirm your suspicions of temporal arteritis as soon as possible, because of the dangers of her developing adverse effects of the condition, such as irreversible and bilateral blindness, if it is not treated immediately that it is detected. Organise blood tests for erythrocyte sedimentation rate (ESR) and C-reactive protein. An ESR above 70 mm/hour will indicate the diagnosis, though such a high ESR and headaches might also be due to a metastatic tumour, myeloma, meningitis or tuberculosis. A normal ESR does not exclude the diagnosis of temporal arteritis but makes it unlikely. A raised C-reactive protein is a non-specific test that indicates the presence of inflammation. A temporal artery biopsy should confirm the diagnosis, although a negative biopsy does not completely exclude giant cell arteritis because of the patchy nature of the arterial condition.

If there were to be any delay in hospital referral and the undertaking of the temporal artery biopsy, you are best to start a high dose of steroids such as 40 mg prednisolone per day, reducing the dose down gradually and titrating against the ESR, over time. A plummeting ESR in response to steroid therapy supports the diagnosis of temporal arteritis. Explain to Mrs Coot that this is a long-term treatment where steroids are gradually reduced over at least two years and maybe as long as five years; and that if she is weaned off steroid medication too quickly her condition is more likely to relapse. Up to a half of patients are able to discontinue steroids within two years of the initial diagnosis.

Migraine

Box 8.4: Case study

Mr Half has come to consult you about his headaches, which he has had off and on since starting work in the local pottery factory 20 years ago when he was 16 years old. Since then he has had an occasional headache but they are becoming more frequent now and he is afflicted about once a week, with headaches lasting for at least eight hours. Sometimes he gets tingling on the left side of his face for an hour or so, affecting his tongue and lips, and usually feels nauseated, occasionally vomiting when his headache is in full flight. Upon enquiry, he admits that he sometimes experiences flashing dots in front of his eyes before the headache starts, which disappear when the headache occurs. His eyesight is fine afterwards and the tingling soon disappears. He is worried about keeping his job as he's missed several days at work this year already because of his headaches.

What issues you should cover

After considering and dismissing non-migraine causes of headache (such as those covered elsewhere in this chapter) you will categorise Mr Half's headaches as migraine from his initial description and from further questioning. The International Headache Society criteria[2,3] are given in Box 8.5 and so you will want to focus your questioning to confirm your preliminary diagnosis of migraine and differentiate between common migraine and classic migraine. It seems as though Mr Half has classic migraine from the symptoms he has described so far.

Box 8.5: International Headache Society criteria (1988)[3]

Migraine without aura (common migraine):
Five or more headache attacks lasting for 4–72 hours with accompanying symptoms of either nausea/vomiting and/or phonophobia or photophobia, with the patient being well between attacks. Pain should have at least two of the following characteristics:

- unilateral
- throbbing
- moderate to severe intensity
- increases with physical activity.

continued overleaf

Migraine with aura (focal or classic migraine):
Two or more headache attacks that have, in addition to the above, at least three of the following characteristics:

- one or more fully reversible aura symptoms indicating focal cerebral cortical and/or brainstem dysfunction
- at least one aura symptom developing gradually over more than four minutes or two or more symptoms occurring in succession
- no aura symptom should last more than one hour
- headache follows aura with a pain-free interval of less than 60 minutes.

Mr Half's symptoms fit with migraine – his neurological symptoms do disappear when he is headache free between attacks. About 7% of men and 20% of women are affected by migraine, although only a small proportion seek help from doctors for it.[4] On average someone with migraine will have three attacks per month and spend five or six hours in bed per attack. Like Mr Half, substantial time is lost from work because of migraine – estimates of average time lost per year are eight days due to absenteeism and 11 days because of reduced efficiency.[4]

You might use the migraine disability assessment questionnaire[5] or the Headache Impact Test[6] to assess the impact of the migraine headaches on Mr Half, or monitor the effectiveness of treatments.

Self-management of migraine

Advice you can give to Mr Half and patients like him includes (adapted from US Headache Consortium guidelines):[4]

- know what the diagnosis of your headache is. Recurrent, disabling headaches are usually migraine headaches
- find a good clinician who understands your problem and is willing to work with you to find appropriate treatment
- tell your doctor how your headache affects your life with any temporary disability
- avoid or reduce factors in your life that trigger your headaches – certain foods, pressures in your life, alcohol, altered sleep patterns, bright lights and hunger
- find appropriate medication for your migraine headaches – the type will depend on the nature and severity of your migraine and range from over the counter to prescription only medication
- do not overuse medication to relieve pain, which might trigger rebound headaches as the initial medication wears off

- have at least two treatment options available – a stronger or 'rescue' medication if the first drug taken is ineffective against a severe attack of migraine
- if one medication for migraine does not work, try another. If the medication does not provide sufficient relief after you have tried it for three attacks, try another type
- ask your doctor about preventive drugs
- use treatments for migraine other than drugs such as biofeedback and relaxation.

You might direct him to useful websites where he can obtain information.[7,8]

Medication for migraine

You are aiming to help Mr Half control his migraine attacks and minimise their impact on his life. Aspirin, non-steroidal anti-inflammatory drugs, and analgesics in combination may be effective for mild to moderate migraine, preferably taken after the migraine attack starts but before the headache develops. Mr Half might already have tried these unsuccessfully. Triptans are an effective treatment for acute migraine attacks of moderate to severe intensity, taken as soon as possible after the headache has started (usually orally, but can be as nasal or subcutaneous formulations). The guidelines recommend that you progress to another medication after at least three treatment failures – so give the drugs a chance.[9]

   Medication you might try where there is evidence that the drug *is* beneficial is:[2]

- aspirin – alone or in combination with metoclopramide, or in combination with paracetamol and caffeine
- eletriptan
- naratriptan
- rizatriptan
- sumatriptan
- zolmitriptan

or where the evidence is that the drug *is likely to be* beneficial:[2]

- diclofenac
- ibuprofen
- naproxen
- tolfenamic acid
- ergotamine derivatives.

Some patients use complementary treatments such as feverfew or acupuncture.

Women who experience focal migraine while taking the combined contra-ceptive pill should find a different method of contraception because of their heightened risk of stroke.

Prophylactic treatment for migraine

If treatment with acute medications is unsatisfactory and he is continuing to get at least two episodes of migraine a month, you might try Mr Half on a prophylactic drug. If he keeps a diary of attacks, he can see if the medication is reducing the frequency of attacks over the next 4–6 weeks. You could switch the type of prophylactic drug at his review if the migraine attacks persist unchanged. You might try a non-cardioselective beta-blocker, such as propranolol, provided he does not also have asthma (as many people with migraine have both). Pizotifen is often successful but weight gain can be a problem. Sodium valproate or amitriptyline are alternative prophylactic treatments.[9]

Follow-up

You could ask Mr Half to keep a headache and event diary and review this with him at follow up, looking for patterns or trends and at the impact the headaches have on his daily life. You can reinforce lifestyle changes, if Mr Half has taken action to reduce triggers to his migraine.

You might try different acute medications if previous ones are not suffi-ciently effective. If prophylactic medication has been successful in reducing the frequency and severity of migraine attacks try tailing it off after about six months.

Collecting data to demonstrate your learning, competence, performance and standards of service delivery

Example cycle of evidence 8.1

- Focus: relationships with patients
- Other relevant focus: clinical care

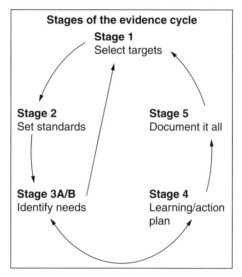

Stages of the evidence cycle

Stage 1
Select targets

Stage 2
Set standards

Stage 5
Document it all

Stage 3A/B
Identify needs

Stage 4
Learning/action plan

Box 8.6: Case study

Mr Port was well known to you because, after several attempts, you had found that sumatriptan controlled his migraine better than any of the other types of medication and he no longer missed days off work as a car salesman. So you were surprised to find him back again complaining that his headaches were back as an everyday event, there when he awoke in the morning. He said that the persistent tingling and numbness in his left arm was making writing difficult as he was left handed.

This is just an example. Keep your task simple. You could choose three or four cycles of evidence to demonstrate your competence each year.

Stage 1: Select your aspirations for good practice

The excellent GP:

- uses clear language appropriate for patients
- gives patients the information they need about their problem in a way they can understand
- provides or arranges investigations or treatment when necessary.

Stage 2: Set the standards for your outcomes

Outcomes might include:

- the way learning is applied
- a learnt skill
- a protocol
- a strategy that is implemented
- meeting recommended standards.

- Good consultation and communication skills with patients that enable patients to be involved in making decisions about their care.
- Early referral of suspected cancer to hospital specialist.

Stage 3A: Identify your learning needs

- Keep a reflective diary where you make notes when you consider there is any possibility of cancer and your degree of confidence in your clinical management and ordering of investigations.
- Review patient case notes when the consultant confirms a diagnosis of cancer: could the patient's cancer have been detected earlier at any point since the initial presentation with associated symptoms or signs?
- Ask colleagues to comment in general, or specifically, on whether patients who have consulted you understand the details you have given them about their illness or condition.

Stage 3B: Identify your service needs

Any of the needs assessment exercises in 3A may also reveal service needs.

- Review patient information materials available to patients with cancer: what leaflets are in the waiting room or your consulting room, what videos are available, what websites can be readily recommended to patients?

- Reflect on whether you know which investigations GPs have open access to, and which require a hospital consultant's request.

Stage 4: Make and carry out a learning and action plan

- Read up on headache and in particular the differentiation between migraine and other serious causes of headache.
- Arrange to join the local neurology consultant for a couple of outpatient sessions to brush up on neurological examination and symptoms and signs giving cause for concern.
- Search for websites on headache and review them for their appropriateness for patients with headache. Print off a list and disseminate it to others in your team or start a practice paper or computer desktop folder of recommended websites for a full range of conditions.

Stage 5: Document your learning, competence, performance and standards of service delivery

- Keep anonymised patients' notes comparing your diagnoses and the hospital consultants' written views/diagnosis.
- Make brief notes of colleagues' perceptions of your ability to explain clinical matters to patients.
- Keep a log of types of investigations available and which you may organise directly with ordering details and locations.
- Keep reflective notes on reading about headache.
- Compile lists of recommended websites.

Box 8.7: Case study continued

You realised straight away that the headaches Mr Port was experiencing were different from his long-standing migraine and that the persistence of the neurological symptoms of tingling and numbness of his left hand were ominous symptoms. You immediately referred Mr Port to the local neurologist. She organised an MRI scan that indicated a space-occupying lesion. Next time you saw Mr Port he was in the midst of a course of radiotherapy for his brain tumour.

Example cycle of evidence 8.2

- Focus: treatment in emergencies
- Other relevant foci: clinical care; working with colleagues; management

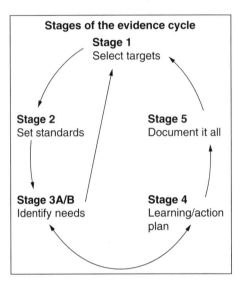

Stages of the evidence cycle

Stage 1
Select targets

Stage 2
Set standards

Stage 5
Document it all

Stage 3A/B
Identify needs

Stage 4
Learning/action
plan

Box 8.8:   Case study

The receptionist puts a call through to you from Mrs Retch, as she is asking for an immediate visit for her 15-year-old daughter. When Mrs Retch described her daughter as having a severe headache with neck pain, and you heard her noisily vomiting in the background, you rushed round to her house, 100 yards away.

This is just an example. Keep your task simple. You could choose three or four cycles of evidence to demonstrate your competence each year.

Stage 1: Select your aspirations for good practice

The excellent GP:

- responds rapidly to emergencies
- works effectively with the emergency services
- makes appropriate judgements about patients who need referral.

Stage 2: Set the standards for your outcomes

Outcomes might include:

- the way learning is applied
- a learnt skill
- a protocol
- a strategy that is implemented
- meeting recommended standards.

- Update the practice protocol for contacting the doctor in emergencies.
- Have an emergency bag maintained with in-date drugs and all essential equipment.

Stage 3A: Identify your learning needs

- Reflect on differential diagnoses for severe headache of abrupt onset and how you might distinguish between subarachnoid haemorrhage, meningitis and acute onset of migraine.
- Compare drug contents of your emergency bag with the list recommended for GP registrars by your course organiser.

Stage 3B: Identify your service needs

Any of the needs assessment exercises in 3A may also reveal service needs.

- Ask members of the practice team if they have any difficulties contacting a doctor in response to a request by a patient for an emergency visit, or they believe that there may be an emergency. Check that the practice protocol for contacting a doctor in an emergency is well known and that the team is satisfied with the contents of the protocol.
- Undertake a significant event audit as a practice team, of one or more cases where there is a delay in visiting a patient with an emergency condition.

Stage 4: Make and carry out a learning and action plan

- Look at the protocols from other practices for contacting a doctor in an emergency and compare them with that in your practice. Revise yours with colleagues as necessary.

- Attend a workshop on headache led by a GPwSI in neurology.
- Spend time thinking through the various actions you would take for common emergencies. Check in books, etc, where you are doubtful that you know exactly how to act, e.g. what dose of drugs to give people of different age groups.

Stage 5: Document your learning, competence, performance and standards of service delivery

- Compare the contents of your emergency bag against that recommended.
- Make notes on the significant event audit and ensuing action plan.
- Develop a revised practice protocol for contacting a doctor in an emergency.
- Keep a record of attendance and participation at the neurology workshop.

Box 8.9:   Case study continued

You rush off on the emergency visit, assuming that any sudden onset of headache reaching its peak in seconds is a subarachnoid haemorrhage until proved otherwise. By the time you arrived at Mrs Retch's house some ten minutes later, her daughter had stopped vomiting but was drowsy and confused. She had no pyrexia or rash and her mother said that her daughter had said that her head had 'exploded' about an hour ago. You arranged an ambulance for her urgent transfer to hospital. Mrs Retch came to see you the following week to report that her daughter had recovered well from her subarachnoid haemorrhage and was waiting to be operated upon in the next few days.

Example cycle of evidence 8.3

- Focus: keeping good records
- Other relevant foci: maintaining good medical practice; prescribing

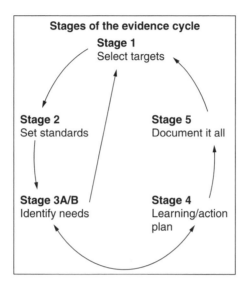

Stages of the evidence cycle

Stage 1
Select targets

Stage 2
Set standards

Stage 5
Document it all

Stage 3A/B
Identify needs

Stage 4
Learning/action
plan

Box 8.10:   Case study

It is Miss Worn's sixth visit to complain about her headaches in the last year, but the first time you have seen her. She tells you she has been to see all your GP colleagues in turn and they have all given her different tablets but nothing seems to work for long. When the tablets wear off the headache is back with a vengeance. You look through her notes to find that she has had very many courses of various analgesics in the last year, some of which had been repeated. She also has had many acute prescriptions overlapping with repeat supplies of analgesics.

This is just an example. Keep your task simple. You could choose three or four cycles of evidence to demonstrate your competence each year.

Stage 1: Select your aspirations for good practice

The excellent GP:

- makes sound management decisions, which are based on good practice and evidence
- records appropriate information for all contacts
- only prescribes treatments that make an effective contribution to the patient's overall management.

Stage 2: Set the standards for your outcomes

> Outcomes might include:
>
> - the way learning is applied
> - a learnt skill
> - a protocol
> - a strategy that is implemented
> - meeting recommended standards.

- An effective repeat prescribing policy that is consistently applied.

Stage 3A: Identify your learning needs

- Keep a reflective diary noting down any concerns about repeat prescribing, of analgesics in particular, about side-effects, overdosage and lack of coherent approach by different GPs in the practice.
- Collect feedback from patients about their management, asking ten consecutive patients with headache e.g. using consultation styles questionnaire.[10]

Stage 3B: Identify your service needs

> Any of the needs assessment exercises in 3A may also reveal service needs.

- Carry out a patient survey or comment form about repeat prescribing and how it works in practice.
- Do a SWOT analysis of repeat prescribing by the practice team with a subsequent action plan to update or revise current practice policy.
- Audit the adherence of the practice team to the repeat prescribing policy in respect of repeat prescribing of analgesics.

Stage 4: Make and carry out a learning and action plan
- Meet up with the pharmaceutical adviser to discuss the repeat prescribing policy and the prescribing of analgesics on acute and repeat bases. Meet the adviser on your own or with practice colleagues after discussing your needs with them.
- Attend an update lecture on headache and reflect on your own part played in patients suffering from chronic headache triggered by overuse of analgesics.
- Arrange a follow-up meeting with other interested people in the practice to discuss the audit and/or SWOT analysis results, the proposed revisions to practice repeat prescribing in general, and the practice protocol for repeat prescribing and concurrent prescribing of various analgesics.

Stage 5: Document your learning, competence, performance and standards of service delivery
- Make reflections in a diary relevant to repeat prescribing in general, and analgesics in particular.
- Collect patient feedback in whichever form you choose.
- Conduct an audit and record the conclusion with the action plan.
- Carry out a SWOT analysis with the action plan.
- Revise your repeat prescribing policy, with a re-audit planned for 12 months' time.

Box 8.11:   Case study continued

Miss Worn takes some convincing about the possible adverse consequences of overuse of analgesics. However, she agrees to give it a go to wean off her present analgesic medication over the following three weeks and try without any analgesic drugs while she is away on holiday. She returns after her holiday, not about her headaches, which are much better if not practically disappeared, but to request medication for her traveller's diarrhoea.

References

1   Risdale L (2003) 'I saw a great star, most splendid and beautiful': headache in primary care. *British Journal of General Practice*. **53**: 182–3.

2   Godlee F (ed.) (2003) *Clinical Evidence*. BMJ Publishing Group, London. www.clinicalevidence.com.

3   Headache Classification Committee of the International Headache Society (1988) Classification and diagnostic criteria for headache disorders, cranial neuralgia and face pain. *Cephalgia*. **8**: 12–96.

4 Moore A, Edwards J, Barden J *et al.* (2003) *Bandolier's Little Book of Pain.* Oxford University Press, Oxford.

5 www.midas-migraine.net.

6 www.amihealthy.com.

7 www.migraine.org.uk.

8 www.migrainetrust.org.

9 Foord-Kelcey G (ed.) (2003) *Guidelines* vol. 20. Medendium Group Publishing Ltd, Berkhamsted.

10 Tate P (2001) *The Doctor's Communication Handbook.* Radcliffe Medical Press, Oxford.

9

Epilepsy

First diagnosis

Box 9.1: Case study

Miss Quaver, a 16-year-old, attends your evening surgery with her mother. That morning her mother had found her in a confused state with blood coming out of her mouth. Her mother had initially thought her daughter's state was a result of recreational drug usage and therefore delayed obtaining medical advice. Miss Quaver denies illicit drug usage. She recalls getting up early and noticed her hands jerked and then she lost consciousness. She remembers noticing her hands jerking on several occasions in last few months, especially if she got up early. On one occasion, she found herself on the bathroom floor having wet herself, but she was so embarrassed she did not confide in her parents.

What issues you should cover

Allow Miss Quaver to tell her story sequentially, and then get an account from her mother. Ask about previous episodes of a similar nature or other curious phenomena, such as myoclonal jerks, olfactory hallucinations, and episodes of déjà vu or dream-like states. Gently probe into her drug and alcohol usage, noting her body language for whether she is being open, although this may be difficult in her mother's presence. Find out about sleep deprivation or stress, e.g. from imminent examinations at school.

Deal with the presenting condition

It is likely that Miss Quaver has had a generalised tonic–clonic epileptic seizure. The morning myoclonic jerks suggest the possibility of a relatively rare form of primary epilepsy called Juvenile Myoclonic Epilepsy (JME).[1] In her age group it would be very unusual for her epilepsy to be secondary to a brain tumour.

It would be reasonable to raise the possibility of epilepsy with Miss Quaver and her mother and to make a referral to a local neurologist. It is probably premature to start an antiepileptic drug at this stage.

Miss Quaver's mother should be advised about what to do if someone has a seizure:

1 remove the person from harm (e.g. proximity to a fire)
2 do not put anything in the patient's mouth
3 put the person in the recovery position as soon as possible. If the seizure (convulsion) lasts more than five minutes, call for paramedics to come via the ambulance service
4 stay with the person after the seizure for at least 20 minutes and reassure them
5 tuck the person up in bed to sleep it off as soon as possible. While the individual is asleep, check him or her at intervals to ensure that the seizure has not started again.

Although it is not relevant in Miss Quaver's case, car drivers should be advised not to drive until an alternative diagnosis has been made or advice sought from the driving licence authorities.

Changing medication

> **Box 9.2:**   Case study
>
> Mr Friendly is a 48-year-old representative for a pharmaceutical company. About 15 years ago, he had had a problem with drinking too much alcohol and had a number of epileptic seizures. He had been banned from driving for a year because of a drink drive conviction. He was started on phenytoin and has been taking it ever since. He has recently started working with a pharmaceutical company that is promoting a new 'wonderful' antiepileptic drug. He has read about the long-term side-effects of phenytoin and wants to change drugs.

What issues you should cover

This consultation will largely revolve around his lifestyle. Find out how secure his job is and how dependent he is on a driving licence. Secondly, try to establish how much alcohol he drinks now.

Ask whether he has had any full or partial seizures in the intervening years. Some partial seizures, such as olfactory hallucinations, may not be recognised by patients as partial attacks. He seems knowledgeable about the long-term complications of phenytoin usage that include:

- gum hypertrophy
- cerebellar atrophy
- peripheral neuropathy
- osteomalacia
- folate deficiency.

Deal with the presenting condition

If the seizures were alcohol related and Mr Friendly is now abstinent from alcohol, or drinks very little, it might be possible to wean him off the phenytoin without substituting another antiepileptic drug, Such a weaning process should be slow, such as at a rate of 100 mg per month. If his lifestyle is dependent on the driving, even substitution with an alternative drug will not guarantee that he remains seizure free and he may be better off with the drug he knows, particularly if the dose and drug levels in the blood are relatively low. You need to advise him that:

- any unexplained loss of consciousness or epileptic seizure is likely to cause a loss of an ordinary driving licence for 12 months
- the driving licence regulators will view any epileptic attack, whether it is partial (just an aura) or generalised, in a similar fashion
- if there is a track record of three years of only nocturnal seizures (when asleep or going to or waking from sleep), it may be possible to hold an ordinary driving licence
- in order to hold a vocational driving licence the person has to be attack free and off medication for 10 years.[2]

Childbearing

Box 9.3: Case study

Miss Swell, a 25-year-old woman, comes to see you, as she is concerned about the medication (valproate) she is taking for her epilepsy that she has had since childhood. She has not had a fit for eight years and now wants to start a family. She wants to know if valproate is 'safe'.

What issues you should cover

Ask Miss Swell about her epilepsy. How many attacks did she have? Did she have any myoclonic jerks? How imminent is her intent to start a family? Is she already pregnant?

Deal with the presenting problem

Discuss the issue of risk and teratogenicity in general. The preliminary results from the UK Epilepsy and Pregnancy Register indicated that around 95% of babies born to women with epilepsy showed no major congenital malformations.[3] Miss Swell is correct to be concerned about the teratogenicity of valproate, as between 5% and 10% of babies born to mothers taking this drug in the first trimester will have an abnormality.[3] If she only had a couple of seizures, she may want to avoid all antiepileptic drugs, at least for the first trimester.

Miss Swell's dependency on the motor car and the risk of her having more seizures will be the determining factors that decide if she is going to substitute another antiepileptic drug, probably lamotrigine, or tail off the valproate. Miss Swell will have to decide for herself what is the right course of action. She may need additional advice from a neurologist, but it is useful to help her to start thinking through the options so she can make a reasoned decision once she is armed with as much information as possible.[4] Start her on 5 mg of folic acid a day, prior to conception. The higher dose of folic acid is to compensate for the possibility of her being folate deficient on her medication, and to protect the foetus against neural tube defects. It would be sensible to ensure her contraception is adequate until conditions have been optimised for the baby she hopes to conceive.

Managing patients with a history of epilepsy

Box 9.4:   Case study

A woman from London has moved to your village and registered as a new patient. Miss Metro is a 35-year-old woman who has a history of endocarditis and an aortic valve replacement. She is on lifelong warfarin and is also taking the oral contraceptive pill. At the time of her endocarditis, she had a single generalised tonic–clonic seizure and was put on phenytoin. She has developed hirsutism and this has been attributed to the phenytoin. As the risk of further seizures is low, she wishes to discontinue the phenytoin.

What issues should be covered

Young people do not often get endocarditis and this suggests that your new patient has a history of intravenous drug usage. You should explore this. Discuss the control of her anticoagulation and her contraceptive needs. As the phenytoin is withdrawn, there will be a reduction in the induction of liver enzymes resulting in increased efficacy of the warfarin and the oral contraceptive pill. You will need to monitor her prothrombin time more closely. Oestrogen-containing contraceptives are contraindicated in women with a history of endocarditis, but she could use a long-acting progestogen method, such as a progestogen-bearing intrauterine system.[5] The phenytoin will need to be withdrawn slowly at a rate of 100 mg a month. You need to bear in mind the important interactions with antiepileptic medications:

- phenytoin, carbamazepine and topiramate are liver enzyme inducers. They reduce the circulating levels of warfarin and hormonal contraceptives
- valproate increases the levels of lamotrigine
- adding lamotrigine to carbamazepine may induce toxic side-effects from the carbamazepine.

Providing a service to people with epilepsy

The ideal outcome for people with epilepsy is for them to be seizure free, with no side-effects from their medication, and leading a normal lifestyle. This is achievable for the majority of patients with epilepsy. However about 20% of patients develop refractory epilepsy and it this group that presents a challenge to healthcare professionals to optimise their quality of life. A good service in primary care to patients with epilepsy would have:

- a database of all patients with epilepsy
- periodic review of patients with intractable epilepsy
- periodic review of patients on older antiepileptic drugs e.g. annually
- members of the primary care team with particular expertise in the management of patients with epilepsy, e.g. a practice nurse and/or a GP
- close links with the local epilepsy liaison nurse and neurosciences services
- sources of information for healthcare professionals and patients (written and online[6]).

Quality indicators in epilepsy

The quality points available in general practice are achievable on a sliding scale, so as you are collecting the data to demonstrate your own competence you are also helping to show that your practice is achieving high standards of care. For many practices, this will be a new area to demonstrate their quality of care. Although this is not a high scoring domain, the four indicators will show that you are improving the care of patients with epilepsy and reducing seizure frequency. The domains are:

- a register of patients receiving drug treatment for epilepsy: 2 points
- 90% of patients over 16 years of age on drug treatment have a seizure frequency recorded in the last 15 months: 4 points
- 90% of patients over 16 years of age on drug treatment have had a medication review in the last 15 months: 4 points
- 70% of patients over 16 years of age on drug treatment have a record that they have been seizure free for 12 months: 6 points.

Most GP software systems have a template for recording the management of epilepsy. You will need to check that the register only includes those patients with a confirmed diagnosis of epilepsy, not those taking antiepileptic medication for pain control. One person in the practice should be responsible for recalling those patients who need an annual review on a rolling programme. Currently there is no Read code for recording freedom from seizures, so you may need to allocate a practice code so that audits can easily retrieve all the information you require. Grounds for excluding patients from the fourth indicator might be a patient on maximum medication who still has poor control, e.g. with severe brain damage, or patients who have unacceptable side-effects with medication.

Principles of use of antiepileptic drugs

The overriding principle in the use of antiepileptic drugs (*see* Figure 9.1 and Table 9.1) is to use the minimum effective dose. Not all people who have seizures automatically require antiepileptic drugs. For example, some people may have infrequent or minor attacks and do not need treatment unless they also drive. Others may have attacks that are not epileptic, or may only have attacks precipitated by conditions such as drinking excess alcohol.

There are a large number of antiepileptic drugs available, so become familiar with some of the more commonly used ones such as phenytoin, carbamazepine, valproate and lamotrigine as well as a couple of the 'new kids on the block', topiramate and levetiracetam. Certain drugs work better in some types of epilepsy (*see* Table 9.1).

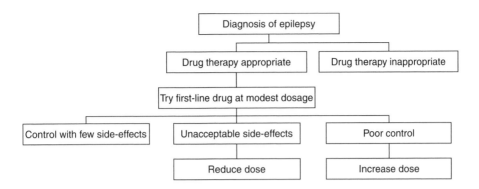

Figure 9.1:   Flow chart for the use of antiepileptic drugs.

Table 9.1:   Antiepileptic drugs and their indications

Drug	Date of introduction	Primary indications Some drugs are also used for other types of epilepsy
Old antiepileptic drugs		
Phenobarbitone	1912	Primary general seizures, focal seizures
Phenytoin	1938	Primary generalised seizures; focal seizures
Carbamazepine	1965	Focal seizures
Sodium valproate	1973	Primary generalised seizures; juvenile myoclonic epilepsy
Newer antiepileptic drugs		
Vigabatrine (Sabril)	1989	Focal seizures
Lamotrigine (Lamictal)	1991	Primary generalised seizures; juvenile myoclonic epilepsy; focal seizures
Gabapentin (Neurontin)	1993	Focal seizures
Topiramate (Topamax)	1994	Primary generalised seizures; juvenile myoclonic epilepsy
Tiagabine (Gabitril)	1994	Focal seizures
Oxcarbamazepine (Trileptal)	1999	Focal seizures
Levetiracetam (Kepra)	2000	Focal seizures

Sudden unexplained death in epilepsy

About 500 people a year die from sudden unexplained death in epilepsy
(SUDEP) in the UK.[7] It is the sudden unexpected death of a person with epilepsy
where there is no alternative explanation such as drowning or trauma. Most
patients are aware that having epilepsy can be dangerous, but telling patients
about SUDEP requires tact and good timing. Epilepsy liaison nurses are
particularly good at imparting this sort of information.[1]

Risk factors for SUDEP are:

- being a young adult male
- poorly controlled epilepsy
- poor compliance with medication
- taking multiple antiepileptic drugs
- frequent changes in medication
- nocturnal seizures
- being alone at the time of the seizure
- suffering generalised tonic–clonic seizures
- having brain damage.

Collecting data to demonstrate your learning, competence, performance and standards of service delivery

Example cycle of evidence 9.1

- Focus: clinical care
- Other relevant foci: working with colleagues; relationships with patients; teaching and training

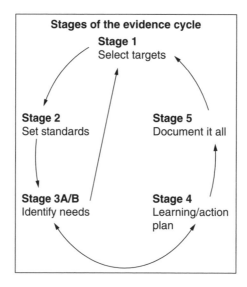

Stages of the evidence cycle

Stage 1
Select targets

Stage 2
Set standards

Stage 5
Document it all

Stage 3A/B
Identify needs

Stage 4
Learning/action plan

Box 9.5: Case study

Mr Sniff has been having 'fainting dos' for the last four years. His parents want to know when he will grow out of them. He is now 17 years old and his parents brought him to see you this time after a particularly nasty event in which he bit his tongue and lost control of his urine. On this occasion, you have a medical student sitting in with you and longer appointment times. You take a fuller history than you might otherwise have done. You take a detailed history of Mr Sniff's fainting attacks initially subjectively from Mr Sniff, then objectively via the eyewitness reports from his parents. You hear that Mr Sniff smells a burnt orange smell before fainting. Mr Sniff has attended several doctors previously with this complaint, but has always been seen urgently, as an extra patient added to the surgery list, and has never been followed up.

This is just an example. Keep your task simple. You could choose three or four cycles of evidence to demonstrate your competence each year.

Stage 1: Select your aspirations for good practice

The excellent GP:

- is prepared to review diagnosis when symptom and clinical course do not seem to fit
- is aware of the several presentations of epilepsy
- refers to another practitioner when indicated
- works with colleagues to monitor and maintain the quality of care provided
- helps to educate other colleagues at all levels.

Stage 2: Set the standards for your outcomes

Outcomes might include:

- the way learning is applied
- a learnt skill
- a protocol
- a strategy that is implemented
- meeting recommended standards.

- Demonstrate your knowledge of the various ways in which epilepsy may present.
- Make appropriate referrals for patients who may have epilepsy.
- Audit changes to practice when best practice has not been shown by you and your colleagues.

Stage 3A: Identify your learning needs

- Carry out a significant event audit of the last patient in whom you made a diagnosis of epilepsy and consider whether there was a delay in diagnosis.
- Keep a reflective diary of patients who present with loss of consciousness, analysing why patients have been put in various diagnostic categories.
- Self-assess your level of knowledge about the various ways in which epilepsy can present.

Stage 3B: Identify your service needs

Any of the needs assessment exercises in 3A may also reveal service needs.

- In patients with an established diagnosis of epilepsy critically re-evaluate the evidence for the diagnosis.
- Review all patients in the practice on antiepileptic medication to check that they are categorised appropriately.
- Review all patients on old-fashioned antiepileptic drugs such as phenytoin or phenobarbitone (these drugs may be entirely appropriate, but a number of patients on long-term antiepileptic drugs do not need drugs at present and may never have had epilepsy).
- Carry out a significant event audit of Mr Sniff's care to establish what changes to the care provided by you and your colleagues are needed.

Stage 4: Make and carry out a learning and action plan

- Read up, or watch a video presentation, on types of epilepsy.
- Prepare for and run a teaching session for medical students assigned to your practice about loss of consciousness.
- Attend a study day on epilepsy supported by the local branch of the British Epilepsy Association.
- Spend a day with an epilepsy liaison nurse.
- Discuss with colleagues how patients with epilepsy are diagnosed in your practice.

- Ask for a constructive critique of your last referral to a consultant neurologist either from the neurologist or from another partner in the practice.

Stage 5: Document your learning, competence, performance and standards of service delivery

- Keep a record of the feedback about your presentation about epilepsy from the medical student and your colleagues.
- Re-audit your patients on antiepilepsy drugs in six months' time.
- Record the critique of your last referral to a consultant neurologist either from the neurologist or from another partner in the practice.
- Repeat your reflective diary of patients presenting with loss of consciousness.
- Re-audit the care of patients who present urgently to determine if your changes have been effective.

Box 9.6: Case study continued

You discuss the possibility with Mr Sniff and his parents that the extra information you have about these attacks suggests that they may not be simple vaso-vagal faints. You suggest referring Mr Sniff for a neurological opinion.

Your local neurologist makes a diagnosis of epilepsy on the basis of your referral letter containing the detailed account of Mr Sniff's symptoms. He is started on carbamazepine and his attacks cease. Further consultations are required to help Mr Sniff deal with the psychological consequences of the diagnosis, but you are both assisted by support from the epilepsy specialist nurse.

You and your colleagues resolve to ask people who are seen urgently with loss of consciousness to write down their account of what happened, and obtain observers' accounts if possible, before returning to discuss the attack in a less hurried appointment than the one made urgently.

Example cycle of evidence 9.2

- Focus: teaching and training
- Other relevant foci: working with colleagues; maintaining good medical practice

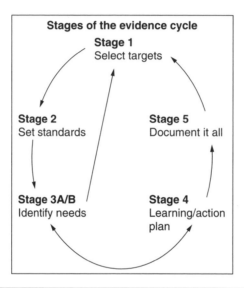

Stages of the evidence cycle

Stage 1
Select targets

Stage 2
Set standards

Stage 5
Document it all

Stage 3A/B
Identify needs

Stage 4
Learning/action plan

Box 9.7:   Case study

You take the lead in your practice team on reproductive health. Following the death in pregnancy of a patient from SUDEP, you agree to organise an in-house training event to raise awareness of the issues. On reflection, the management of the patient was good, but her death has shaken everyone up.

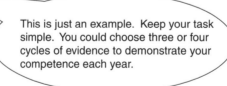

This is just an example. Keep your task simple. You could choose three or four cycles of evidence to demonstrate your competence each year.

Stage 1: Select your aspirations for good practice

The excellent GP:

- understands the health needs of women in their reproductive years who have epilepsy

- helps to educate other colleagues at all levels
- respects the skills and contributions of colleagues
- ensures that the practice team can deliver the care of women in their reproductive years who have epilepsy
- joins in with reviews and audits of standards and performance of the team, and with any steps to remedy deficiencies.

Stage 2: Set the standards for your outcomes

Outcomes might include:

- the way learning is applied
- a learnt skill
- a protocol
- a strategy that is implemented
- meeting recommended standards.

- Demonstrate that the care of women in their reproductive years who have epilepsy is carried out in line with best practice.
- The practice protocol for reviewing patients with epilepsy is in line with best practice.

Stage 3A: Identify your learning needs

- Self-assess what you know about:
  - the teratogenicity of antiepileptic drugs
  - the effects of antiepileptic drugs on fertility
  - interactions between antiepileptic and contraceptive drugs
  - SUDEP.
- Use your reflective diary to record how and what you discuss with patients in the reproductive age group who are taking antiepileptic drugs.

Stage 3B: Identify your service needs

Any of the needs assessment exercises in 3A may also reveal service needs.

- Ask all members of the primary care team to identify what learning needs they have in the areas identified in Stage 3A.

- Invite your local epilepsy liaison nurse to review the systems of care you have for women with epilepsy.
- Review the records of all women of childbearing age who are taking antiepileptic drugs and look for evidence that the team have considered reproductive needs and teratogenicity.

Stage 4: Make and carry out a learning and action plan

- Devise practice protocols for managing women with epilepsy in conjunction with the local epilepsy liaison nurse.
- Have separate protocols for managing the special requirements of young women for contraceptive and pregnancy care.
- If shortfalls are identified, consider if these are best met by addressing training needs within the primary care team or by instituting special arrangements for this at-risk group.
- Plan the in-house learning event around the learning needs established in Stage 3.

Stage 5: Document your learning, competence, performance and standards of service delivery

- Document the audit of the use of valproate in women in their reproductive years, the changes proposed and the date set for re-audit.
- Record findings from the evaluation from the in-house learning event.
- Keep the updated protocols for the care of women with epilepsy in their reproductive years.

Box 9.8:   Case study continued

The audit of women on antiepileptic drugs identified patients who were taking particularly teratogenic antiepileptic drugs. One patient was changed to an alternative drug and another improved the reliability of her contraception following the changes proposed. Following the in-house learning event, the team feel much more confident about managing women with epilepsy in the reproductive years and team morale has improved.

Example cycle of evidence 9.3

- Focus: relationships with patients
- Other relevant foci: clinical care; working with colleagues; probity

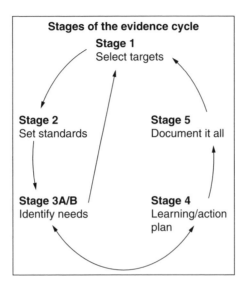

Box 9.9:   Case study

Mr Rule, a patient in the practice with well controlled epilepsy, has a car crash in which fortunately no one was hurt. There is no written evidence that Mr Rule had been advised of his responsibilities with regard to the driving licence authorities.

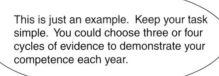

This is just an example. Keep your task simple. You could choose three or four cycles of evidence to demonstrate your competence each year.

Stage 1: Select your aspirations for good practice

The excellent GP:

- understands the driving licence regulations in relation to episodes of loss of consciousness and epilepsy

- gives patients the information they need with regard to safety and legal responsibilities.

Stage 2: Set the standards for your outcomes

Outcomes might include:

- the way learning is applied
- a learnt skill
- a protocol
- a strategy that is implemented
- meeting recommended standards.

- Develop a guideline, agreed with colleagues, on how patients with a potential diagnosis of epilepsy are advised about the driving regulations.
- Agree with colleagues how this information is recorded in the patient record.

Stage 3A: Identify your learning needs

- Self-assess your knowledge of the driving licence regulations and check against the current regulations.[2]
- Search for suitable information leaflets. You might use (with their permission) one written by another practice.[8]

Stage 3B: Identify your service needs

Any of the needs assessment exercises in 3A may also reveal service needs.

- Circulate a questionnaire in the practice to establish what gaps exist in the team's knowledge about the driving regulations.
- Carry out a record search of ten patients recently diagnosed with epilepsy, for any mention of a discussion or information given about the driving licence regulations.

Stage 4: Make and carry out a learning and action plan

- Undertake a short in-house learning event about the legal consequences of a potential or actual diagnosis of epilepsy on drivers. Use the information

gathered from the 'gap analysis' in the first point of 3B and the record search in the second point of 3B.
- Devise a short questionnaire to record the answers after you have given the information leaflet to patients with epilepsy. Collect the feedback for use in your presentation for the in-house learning event.

Stage 5: Document your learning, competence, performance and standards of service delivery

- Keep the evaluation of the in-house learning event with the notes of the discussion points.
- Record the method agreed with colleagues of recording that information about the driving licence regulations has been given.
- Keep a record of the review of the records of any newly diagnosed patient in the next 12 months to look for evidence of information with regard to driving licences being imparted.
- Keep a copy of the leaflet relating to epilepsy and driving that has been handed out.
- Keep a copy of the feedback from patients on their understanding of the regulations and what actions they should take after reading the leaflet.

Box 9.10:   Case study continued

The in-house learning event induced a lively debate about the legal duty of a doctor or nurse to inform the DVLA if they knew that a patient with epilepsy was driving and the ethical duty of confidentiality. Most patients found the leaflet helpful in clarifying what actions they needed to take and whether their driving was restricted. A few were angry about what they regarded as unnecessary restrictions. The record review showed that after 12 months all newly diagnosed patients had a record that the doctor or nurse had discussed the leaflet. The team had given all patients a copy or tape of the leaflet, or had arranged for the leaflet to be translated for those who could not read English.

Example cycle of evidence 9.4

- Focus: clinical care
- Other relevant foci: relationships with patients; working with colleagues; teaching and training

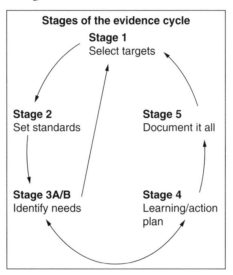

Stages of the evidence cycle

Stage 1
Select targets

Stage 2
Set standards

Stage 5
Document it all

Stage 3A/B
Identify needs

Stage 4
Learning/action plan

Box 9.11: Case study

Mrs Wonder, a 25-year-old patient, has become pregnant. This was a surprise to Mrs Wonder and her husband, as she conscientiously took her combined oral contraceptive pill as well as her carbamazepine for her epilepsy. However, they had planned to start a family in the near future and Mrs Wonder is delighted to be pregnant.

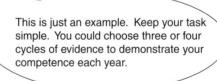

This is just an example. Keep your task simple. You could choose three or four cycles of evidence to demonstrate your competence each year.

Stage 1: Select your aspirations for good practice

The excellent GP:

- has knowledge of important drug interactions with antiepileptic medications

- keeps patients informed of the more important interactions
- helps to educate other colleagues at all levels.

Stage 2: Set the standards for your outcomes

Outcomes might include:

- the way learning is applied
- a learnt skill
- a protocol
- a strategy that is implemented
- meeting recommended standards.

- Ensure that a warning message appears on the prescribing screen when combined oral contraceptives are prescribed to patients taking drugs that are enzyme inducers.
- Ensure that patients are informed about possible interactions when taking drugs that are enzyme inducers.

Stage 3A: Identify your learning needs

- Self-assess your knowledge by reviewing the interactions of the commonly used antiepileptic drugs.[9]
- Carry out a significant event audit on a patient, e.g. one who had had frequent irregular bleeding, and unnecessary investigations, while taking several types of hormone replacement therapy, because of failure to recognise the enzyme enhancement activity of the carbamazepine she was also taking.

Stage 3B: Identify your service needs

Any of the needs assessment exercises in 3A may also reveal service needs.

- Review the electronic prescribing system in use and the identification of potential interactions with antiepileptic drugs.
- Use a quiz at a practice meeting to identify any learning needs with regard to interactions between antiepileptic drugs.
- Obtain feedback from ten patients on enzyme-inducing preparations about their awareness of possible interactions with other drugs.

Stage 4: Make and carry out a learning and action plan

- Discuss with the local epilepsy liaison nurse the drug interactions that cause the most problems in clinical practice and obtain suitable information to give to patients.
- Prepare for and run a teaching session on the interactions of commonly used antiepileptic drugs. Repeat the quiz for your practice team two weeks after the session.
- Find out how to add an interaction alert to the prescribing module on the computer.

Stage 5: Document your learning, competence, performance and standards of service delivery

- Keep the results of the quiz completed by those attending the teaching session before and after the training session.
- Test and record the addition of the interaction warning on the prescribing module.
- Record the information supplied to patients about possible drug interactions.

Box 9.12:   Case study continued

The quiz reveals that some members of the practice team have been unsure about interactions between antiepileptic drugs as well as between antiepileptic drugs and other drugs used to treat patients. More questions are answered correctly after the in-house session. The prescribing alert works well and the practice team agrees to audit the number of patients on combined oral contraceptives and drugs that are enzyme inducers in 12 months' time, to ensure that prescribers are not ignoring the risks.

References

1   Baddeley L and Ellis SJ (2001) *Epilepsy: a team approach to effective management.* Butterworth-Heinemann, Oxford.

2   UK Driving Licence Regulations for Neurological Conditions www.dvla.gov.uk /at_a_glance/ch1_neurological.htm (accessed August 2003).

3   Morrison P (On behalf of the UK Epilepsy and Pregnancy Register) Malformation rates in offspring of mothers in the UK Epilepsy and Pregnancy Register: results from a prospective 7 year study 1996–2002. www.faseb.org/genetics/ashg02s/ f171.htm.

4   Northern Fetal and Maternal Medicine Group: Epilepsy and pregnancy guidelines
     www.ncl.ac.uk/nfmmg/guidelines/epilepsy%20guide.htm (accessed November
     2003).

5   Wakley G and Chambers R (2002) *Sexual Health Matters in Primary Care*. Radcliffe
     Medical Press, Oxford.

6   www.epilepsy.org.uk.

7   British Epilepsy Association. Sudden Unexpected Death in Epilepsy www.epilepsy.
     org.uk/info/sudep.html (accessed August 2003).

8   Smith B, Watson J, Cheek B *et al*. Well Close Square Surgery, Berwick-upon-Tweed.
     Epilepsy: the UK law www.wellclosesquare.co.uk/pal/epilepsy/epillaw.htm (accessed
     August 2003).

9   Joint Formulary Committee (2003) *British National Formulary*. British Medical
     Association and Royal Pharmaceutical Society, London. www.bnf.org.

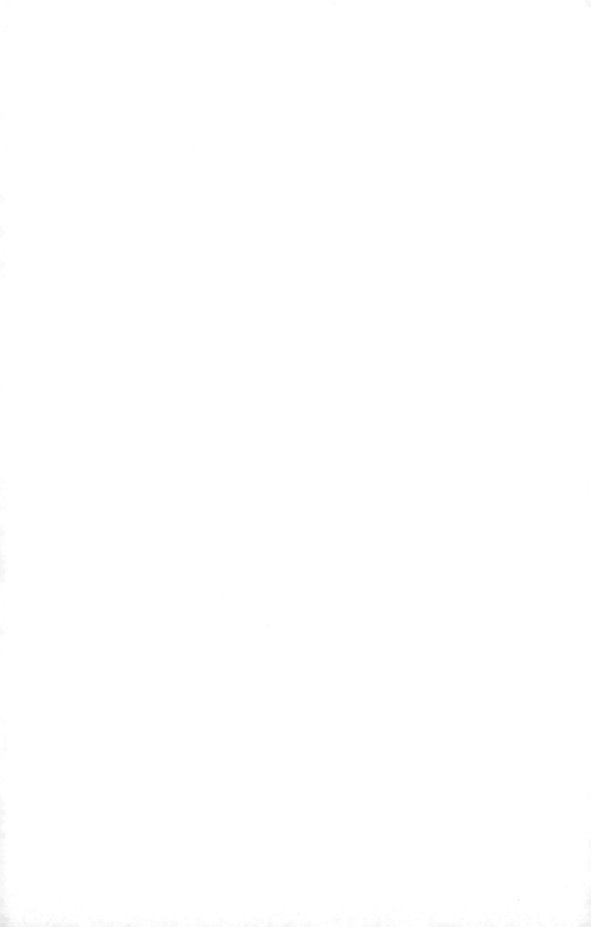

10

Chronic painful conditions

Box 10.1:   Case study

Your GP registrar brings some difficult cases to a tutorial with you. The common theme for all three is that the patient is suffering from chronic pain, which is proving difficult to control over time. The three cases are a 70-year-old man with trigeminal neuralgia, a 75-year-old woman complaining of painful cramps and restless legs at night, and a 60-year-old woman whose post-herpetic neuralgia is poorly controlled.

What issues you should cover

Sociocultural factors, age, the type of painful stimulus, genetic makeup and other factors all combine to affect someone's perception of pain. Gender can be a factor too – men have been shown to have a higher threshold and tolerance to pain in research experiments.[1] Women develop chronic pain disorders more frequently than men and tend to describe pain that is more diffuse. Researchers are investigating the possibility that men and women react differently to some pain-relieving drugs.[1]

Pain is commonly reported. In one study about half of respondents described having pain or discomfort that persisted continuously or intermittently for longer than three months.[2] One third of the 25–34 year olds in this study reported such pain compared to around two-thirds of over-65 year olds.

Pain is very disabling. In Scotland, one study showed that the pain experienced by a quarter of people with chronic pain was highly disabling and at least moderately limiting to their daily lives.[2]

Discuss the nature of chronic pain with patients. They often believe that chronic pain is the same as acute pain, only present all the time. Explain that acute pain is a danger signal that something is wrong. Chronic pain tells you that something has been wrong in the past and the nerves have become used to passing that signal onto the brain. Many people are unwilling to take adequate pain relief for chronic pain because they think they will not be able to receive acute pain warning signals. They need to be aware that they can relieve chronic pain with analgesics but still be able to feel the acute pain of, for example, cutting themselves on the edge of a tin, or pulling a muscle during over-exertion. Beliefs about how chronic pain happens often lead people into inactivity. They avoid anything that might cause the pain in the short term instead of increasing their activity to improve muscle strength and co-ordination and stretch tight scar tissue to decrease the pain in the long term. Taking enough pain relief to prevent the emergence of pain, that is, pro-phylactically and not just in response to pain, reduces the passage of the pain messages along the nerves and helps to prevent the nerves becoming 'accustomed to passing that message'. Established pain leads to structural and neurochemical changes in the central nervous system that consolidate the pattern of pain. Taking enough pain relief also permits the graduated and frequent activity that improves chronic pain.

Measuring pain

Measuring the extent of pain that someone is experiencing involves attempting to quantify their description. Doctors and others have used visual analogue scales in an attempt to quantify pain or other measurement scales such as the McGill Pain Questionnaire (MPQ).[3,4] The short form MPQ consists of 15 descriptive words that are rated according to the intensity and quality of pain. Those using the questionnaire indicate the location of their pain on a paper drawing of their body. It is difficult to apply the MPQ if the patient's perception of pain is constantly varying in terms of its site and intensity. A visual analogue scale is quicker to use, as the patient simply makes a vertical mark on a horizontal line, indicating the intensity of the pain according to the nearness of the mark to the ends of the horizontal line, labelled as nil or extreme pain.

The Pain Society has produced a series of pain scales to assist doctors and other healthcare staff in assessing pain in people for whom English is not their first language. The scales are produced in 16 different languages and can be downloaded from the Internet.[5]

Approaches to chronic pain

Interventions that are available for chronic pain management are presented in Box 10.2. If conventional analgesics relieve chronic pain to an adequate extent with no or with tolerable side-effects, then there is little reason to use other interventions described in Box 10.2 except in accordance with patient preference.

If analgesics are ineffective or cause intolerable side-effects, then the other methods described in Box 10.2 should be considered after checking that the correct analgesics are being given in the correct dose by the correct route at the correct time.[2]

Box 10.2:   Treatment methods for the relief of chronic pain[2]

- Analgesics:
  - conventional medication; ranging from paracetamol and non-steroidal anti-inflammatory drugs (NSAIDs) to morphine-like drugs
  - pain-modulating drugs – antidepressant, anticonvulsant and others
- Block nerve transmission:
  - reversible – e.g. local anaesthetic +/– steroid
  - irreversible – nerve destruction e.g. by neurolysis or radiofrequency
- Alternatives
  - stimulators e.g. transcutaneous electrical nerve stimulation
  - acupuncture
  - hypnosis
  - psychological techniques

Paracetamol

Paracetamol is widely used both purchased over the counter and prescribed by health professionals. Its short action leads to breakthrough pain unless it is taken four times daily and it deals inadequately with night pain. It has little anti-inflammatory action. It is often combined with weak opiates in fixed dose combinations.

Aspirin

Aspirin is an effective pain reliever with good anti-inflammatory properties but is limited by its side-effects, especially those of gastrointestinal haemorrhage, in effective dosages for chronic pain.

Non-steroidal anti-inflammatory drugs

NSAIDs are particularly useful when pain has an inflammatory component. Like aspirin, the risk of bleeding, the development of gastrointestinal ulceration, retention of sodium, hypertension and oedema limit their usefulness. They may trigger bronchospasm in susceptible people. Although selective cox-2 inhibitors may be less likely to cause gastrointestinal ulceration and bleeding, they are only safer, not completely safe.

Combination therapy

Using combination therapy may permit lower doses of each agent that may be better tolerated. A combination of NSAIDs with paracetamol may allow control of pain not managed by higher doses of either alone. NSAIDs may be better tolerated if combined with a gastro-protective agent like a proton pump inhibitor.

Opioids

Opioids may induce physical and psychological dependence in people who are not in pain but such dependence does not appear to happen to people who receive them for pain relief. Opiates cause constipation, sometimes urinary retention, and in larger doses may depress respiration and cause drowsiness, confusion, nausea and vomiting, urticaria and pruritus.

The dose is titrated against the extent of pain and increased as the patient's pain increases unless there are intolerable side-effects. Give opioids regularly without waiting for the pain to return.

Codeine, dihydrocodeine, and dextropropoxyphene are weak opiates often used in fixed dose combinations with paracetamol. It may be easier to titrate the dose using the drugs separately to a level where pain is controlled, before choosing a suitable combination. Strong opiates, such as morphine and fentanyl, are very useful for severe continuous pain. They can be combined with NSAIDs for control of severe pain with inflammation e.g. bone pain. They can be given in sustained release oral formulations or delivered by alternative routes such as sublingual, transdermal, by suppository, by subcutaneous infusion or occasionally by an epidermal route (together with a local anaesthetic).[2] Using a slow release formulation helps to prevent breakthrough pain occurring. Prescribe strong opiates with a stimulant laxative to prevent constipation.

Pain modulating drugs

Amitriptyline is used for pain relief at lower doses than those used in depression, e.g. 10–50 mg, but may still cause problems with a dry mouth, sleepiness and constipation. Other antidepressant medication can also be tried if amitriptyline is not tolerated. Anticonvulsant drugs are used in similar doses for providing analgesia as for controlling fits. Carbamazepine 100 mg three times daily titrating up to 1 g daily is useful for stabbing pain like trigeminal neuralgia, but drowsiness, dizziness, constipation and unsteadiness limit its usefulness at higher doses. Gabapentin 100 mg to 800 mg three times daily is increasingly being used for neuropathic pain and headache. Side-effects of gabapentin also include drowsiness, dizziness, and unsteadiness as well as arthralgia, dysarthria, amnesia, fatigue and weight changes, leucopaenia and purpura. Antidepressants should be tried first as they may cause fewer side-effects than anticonvulsants.[2] Other drugs that are sometimes tried include clonidine and other alpha-2 adrenergic agonists, baclofen and ketamine.

Transcutaneous electrical nerve stimulation

Transcutaneous electrical nerve stimulation (TENS) involves electrodes being placed on the skin and different electrical pulse rates being used to stimulate the affected area at different intensities. The electrodes need to be applied for at least an hour at a time. The intensity of delivery of the high-frequency pulses is sufficiently low to avoid muscle contractions. The theory behind the way it works is that when the spinal cord is bombarded with impulses from the TENS machine then it is distracted from transmitting the pain signals from the person's affected painful area. Evidence of benefits for its use are more clear cut for some conditions than others. It is likely to be beneficial for dysmenorrhoea and neck pain, but is of unknown effectiveness for low back pain and sciatica or chronic pain in general.[2,6–8]

Acupuncture

Acupuncture is needle puncture of the skin at the site of traditional 'meridian' acupuncture sites or trigger points relating to the affected painful area(s). The needles are then stimulated manually or electrically. Most of the trials undertaken in relation to the use of acupuncture have been too small to provide conclusive evidence of its efficacy in chronic pain relief. Most high-quality studies have shown either no benefit or that acupuncture was worse than the controls with which it was compared. Research studies which used methods of investigation ranked as 'low quality' appeared to find that acupuncture had a better treatment effect than research studies where the methods were classified as 'high quality'.[2]

Psychological treatment

Psychological treatment can be helpful if patterns of response have not become too entrenched. Learning to live with the pain, learning to ignore it and carry on with activities despite the pain can be very valuable but patients may need considerable support to achieve this shift in attitude. Group therapy, well facilitated, can help some patients to come to terms with the disability imposed by the pain and become less fearful and more active. Others may need individual therapy, which is in short supply in the NHS. Depression is a frequent accompaniment to chronic pain. Specific cognitive behavioural therapy and sometimes antidepressants may be required, but chronic pain sufferers are often resentful of efforts to treat their understandable depression and hopelessness, fearing that the health professional thinks the pain is imaginary or feigned. Some patients may find that learning self-hypnosis techniques can help to control the pain, especially during exacerbations or when trying to increase activity.

Trigeminal neuralgia

Box 10.3:   Case study

Mr Lance described the pain on the left side of his face as sharp and stabbing like an electric shock. He had had the pain for a few weeks. It had started out of the blue and the attacks seemed to start for no reason, although sometimes washing his face or brushing his teeth could trigger it. The pain lasted about a minute when it came and he reckoned that he had about 50 episodes per day. The pain was so intense that it stopped him in his tracks or occasionally woke him up from sleep. In all his 70 years he had never known pain like it.

What issues you should cover

Trigeminal neuralgia is an intense pain in the distribution of one or more branches of the fifth cranial nerve, the trigeminal nerve. The pain lasts for between a few seconds and two minutes at a time. The episodes of pain generally occur during the day and not at night. Some people have hundreds of attacks a day while others can go for years between attacks. There are reports of trigeminal neuralgia becoming more severe, with shorter remissions and being less responsive to treatment over time. In general it is people over 50 years old who suffer from it. Some people believe that it is triggered by an ectopic artery in contact with the entry of the trigeminal nerve root in the brainstem. The cause is unknown in most cases. People with multiple sclerosis may develop trigeminal neuralgia at a young age and it is more common in women with hypertension.[9]

You will examine Mr Lance to check that there is no other cause for his facial pain such as dental pain. The episodic nature of the pain and the history of provoking the pain by washing and brushing his teeth are a classical history in trigeminal neuralgia.

Carbamazepine reduces the severity and frequency of the paroxysms of pain. Start at 100 mg one to two times daily, increasing up to a dosage of 200 mg three to four times a day.[10] Adverse effects can include rashes, drowsiness, dizziness, constipation and ataxia. In one study, more than two-thirds of people benefited initially from taking carbamazepine for trigeminal neuralgia, but by 5–16 years later, about half required additional treatments.

Pimozide is a cardiotoxic drug that has been used to treat trigeminal neuralgia that proved refractory to carbamazepine, but its use is restricted because of its toxicity and association with sudden death.[9] Other drugs that have been used to treat trigeminal neuralgia that are of unknown effectiveness include: baclofen, lamotrigine, tizanidine, phenytoin, clonazepam, sodium valproate, gabapentin and levetiracetam.[9]

Other types of treatments that are tried include: nerve blocks, acupuncture, alcohol injection, radiofrequency thermocoagulation, injection of phenol and laser treatment – over affected or trigger areas. There is no evidence of effectiveness for any of these approaches.[9]

Box 10.4: Case study continued

Mr Lance is one of the lucky ones, and responds well to carbamazepine. The episodes of pain are completely controlled at a dose of 200 mg three times a day.

Restless legs (Ekbom's syndrome)

Box 10.5: Case study

Miss Fidget has come to consult you because of the aching and tingling she gets in her legs whenever she rests in a chair or lies in bed. She complains that the cramps in her legs at night in bed are so severe that they keep her awake. Moving her legs does relieve the aching. She wants some assistance in controlling the pains in her legs and helping her to sleep better.

Restless legs syndrome usually presents in middle or old age. One in 20 of the population suffer from it to a greater or lesser degree. The restlessness feeling gives the sufferer an urge to move their legs, and subsequent movement relieves the aching symptoms. Symptoms are usually worse at night. Some people also describe involuntary jerking of their legs when they are dropping off to sleep. Miss Fidget has a typical presentation.

What issues you should cover

Most cases of restless legs syndrome are idiopathic. Rule out any other diagnosis which might be associated with, or the underlying cause of, the aching limbs or involuntary twitching. When you examine a patient like Miss Fidget, think of the possibilities of Parkinson's disease, pregnancy, sensory neuropathy (especially that secondary to uraemia or diabetes), side-effects of medication, iron deficiency and rheumatoid arthritis. If any of these conditions were to blame, you would take appropriate action, instigating treatment or altering medication, etc. If there is no underlying condition, you should find that the physical examination is normal.

You would reassure Miss Fidget and explain that her restless legs syndrome had no serious underlying cause, but is likely to be with her for the rest of her life. You might advise her to avoid caffeine or alcohol or stop smoking if any of these are relevant to her lifestyle. She could try hot or cold baths or rubbing her legs. You would check that she has a reasonably nutritious diet and encourage her to take regular exercise. She might get further information about how she can help herself from the Restless Legs Syndrome Foundation or the Ekbom Support Group.[11,12]

If self-help measures fail and her sleep is sufficiently disturbed or Miss Fidget cannot tolerate the symptoms, you might try a benzodiazepine such as diazepam or temazepam as an intermittent therapy to avoid tolerance or dependency. In a refractory case, you might prescribe an anticonvulsant such as clonazepam, gabapentin or sodium valproate, or consider dopaminergic drugs, although you would have to discuss these options with Miss Fidget as they are not licensed for the restless legs syndrome.[13-15]

Post-herpetic neuralgia

Box 10.6:   Case study

You saw Mrs Belt a couple of months ago when she presented with shingles. By the time she came to see you she had had the zoster rash on the left side of her mid-trunk for about two weeks and was worried that it was not clearing up. At that time, the pain she was experiencing was along the line of the fifth thoracic nerve and there were still crops of vesicles with scabs on, over the area. You decided then that it was too late to institute treatment with an antiviral agent. Now she is still complaining of persistent intense pain and itchiness over the site where the rash had been.

Post-herpetic neuralgia is pain that sometimes follows an acute infection with herpes zoster and the healing of the associated rash. Herpes zoster (shingles) is more common in people over 50 years old. Eleven in 1000 people over 80 years old each year will have a herpes zoster infection.[16] Subsequent neuralgia is more likely the older the person is when they suffer from shingles. About a third of those aged over 80 years develop post-herpetic neuralgia.

Herpes zoster is an acute infection caused by the activation of a latent varicella zoster virus in people who have been rendered vulnerable from a previous attack of chickenpox. It affects the sensory ganglia and the areas of the body they serve.

Neuropathic pain post-herpes zoster infection or from diabetes mellitus is often associated with depression. Treatments for which there is good evidence of pain relief are gabapentin or a tricyclic antidepressant such as amitriptyline.[16] Start gabapentin at 300 mg per day, increased daily until there is sufficient pain relief, up to a maximum of 1.8 g per day.[10] Amitriptyline could be started at 10–25 mg at night, and increased up to 75 mg depending on response.[10] Another option is a topical local anaesthetic preparation such as the cream, capsaicin 0.75%, applied three to four times per day, after the herpes zoster lesions have healed – though the evidence for benefit is uncertain.[2]

You could encourage Mrs Belt to understand the cause and effects of her neuropathic pain from self-help materials.[17]

Box 10.7:   Case study continued

Three months later, Mrs Belt's sister developed the pain and rash of herpes zoster, also on her trunk. Mrs Belt encouraged her sister to consult you as soon as the first few vesicles erupted. You were able to prescribe famciclovir 250 mg three times daily for seven days, as she had presented within 72 hours of the onset of the rash.[10] Two months later, she felt well, her rash had cleared and she was no longer experiencing pain over the area where the shingles had been.

Collecting data to demonstrate your learning, competence, performance and standards of service delivery

Example cycle of evidence 10.1

- Focus: relationships with patients
- Other relevant focus: clinical care

Box 10.8:   Case study

The pain that Mrs Wrack is experiencing from her osteoarthritis seems unrelenting. She has been on a waiting list for a knee joint replacement for several months and the pain is so severe that she has difficulty getting about in and outside her house. Being the main carer for her husband who has multiple sclerosis compounds Mrs Wrack's problem. Mrs Wrack thinks that using her knee over the years to stabilise her husband when helping him to dress and move from his bed has caused the osteoarthritis.

This is just an example. Keep your task simple. You could choose three or four cycles of evidence to demonstrate your competence each year.

Stage 1: Select your aspirations for good practice

The excellent GP:

- is up to date with developments in clinical practice and regularly reviews his or her knowledge and performance
- only prescribes treatments that make an effective contribution to the patient's overall management
- accompanies referrals with the information needed by the specialist to make an appropriate and efficient evaluation of the patient's problem.

Stage 2: Set the standards for your outcomes

Outcomes might include:

- the way learning is applied
- a learnt skill
- a protocol
- a strategy that is implemented
- meeting recommended standards.

- Develop a treatment schedule for chronic pain relief.
- Conduct an audit of outcomes of patient referrals for conditions with associated chronic pain, including the patients' perspectives, in line with intended practice.

Stage 3A: Identify your learning needs

- Write down your current approach to chronic pain management for patients with and without cancer, as a flow diagram and compare with a published algorithm of best practice.[2]
- Carry out a survey of patients whom you have treated for chronic pain to determine the extent of pain relief and limitations of daily activities. You might identify ten consecutive patients from requests for repeat prescribing of analgesics or those consulting you as follow ups for pain relief.
- Focus on Mrs Wrack's case and review the original referral letter to see if her home circumstances and caring responsibilities were described to enable the specialist to prioritise her case.

Stage 3B: Identify your service needs

Any of the needs assessment exercises in 3A may also reveal service needs.

- Audit the repeat prescribing of opiates or NSAIDs by asking 20 patients to attend for review of their medication. Find out how long it is since the patient was reviewed, the extent of the pain relief, the existence of any side-effects, and what pain-relieving approaches other than medication have been tried.
- Review the length of time patients with chronic pain are waiting for treatment by others: by a physiotherapist, during the stages in referral to an orthopaedic surgeon and for joint replacement, what equipment is prescribed e.g. a

TENS machine, and the waiting time for an initial appointment at pain clinic. Consider what you might have done to speed any of these processes including supplying evidence to your PCO to influence the commissioning process.

Stage 4: Make and carry out a learning and action plan

- Read up about best practice in relieving chronic pain and the evidence for the various interventions.[2]
- Attend a couple of sessions at the local pain clinic and learn which patients would benefit from being referred and the interventions used in the clinic. Build links with pain clinic staff to enable you to telephone for advice in the future.
- Compose a treatment policy relating to chronic pain relief in general and for various common conditions. Discuss it at the second session at the pain clinic with the specialist in charge.
- Run an educational session at the practice for other GPs, practice nurses, attached physiotherapists, district nurses and any others with an interest, to share patients' views and present the draft treatment policy for discussion, before accepting it as a practice team.
- Discuss how the agreed treatment policy can be implemented with key people in the practice team and decide what shortfalls there are in terms of resources (e.g. availability of equipment or therapy or over-long referral routes) and liaise with the PCO about unmet needs.

Stage 5: Document your learning, competence, performance and standards of service delivery

- Compare your algorithm of chronic pain relief with best practice.
- Keep the results from the patients' survey of the extent of pain relief.
- Keep the referral letter about Mrs Wrack, appropriately anonymised for your portfolio, and your comments on additional information you might have added that would have helped her case to be prioritised.
- Keep the results of an audit of repeat prescribing of analgesics.
- Review the outcomes of referrals of patients with chronic pain.
- Make notes on best practice from reading.
- Make notes on key learning points from sitting in at the pain clinic.
- Keep a copy of the agreed practice treatment policy for chronic pain.
- Keep a copy of the letter to the PCO detailing shortfalls in provision of treatment for patients with chronic pain.

Box 10.9: Case study continued

The PCO used the information you gathered about the inadequacy of resources for prompt management of patients with chronic pain, to review the effectiveness of the referral pathway. The review group included those representing orthopaedic surgery, the pain clinic, allied health professionals in primary care and several patients who had recently been through the system. This resulted in investment of additional resources at all stages and the evaluation of the changes continues.

Example cycle of evidence 10.2

- Focus: if things go wrong
- Other relevant focus: keeping good records

Box 10.10: Case study

When you came into work today there is a message for you from one of your GP colleagues that one of your patients, Mrs Board, has been admitted as an emergency with a severe haematemesis and she is in a bad way. You see from her computer records that she has been taking NSAIDs for two to three years for her chronic back pain. The message from your colleague has been pinned to the paper medical record, which was taken out on the home visit and then left on your desk. You flick through the hospital letters and, to your horror, you see that she has an old history of a gastric ulcer, which was not considered when she was started on her NSAIDs.

This is just an example. Keep your task simple. You could choose three or four cycles of evidence to demonstrate your competence each year.

Stage 1: Select your aspirations for good practice

The excellent GP:

- contacts the patient soon after it is apparent that a mistake has occurred
- tells the patient what has happened and how it can be put right
- co-operates with any investigation arising from a complaint.

Stage 2: Set the standards for your outcomes

Outcomes might include:

- the way learning is applied
- a learnt skill
- a protocol
- a strategy that is implemented
- meeting recommended standards.

- Record how the practice team learns from a mistake to minimise a recurrence.
- Revise the practice protocol for prescribing of NSAIDs in line with recommended practice.

Stage 3A: Identify your learning needs

- Undertake a significant event audit of Mrs Board's case with other GPs responsible for repeat prescribing in your practice.
- Discuss the process for Mrs Board or a relative lodging a complaint with the practice manager and defence society so that you are ready for anything and know how to respond and be fair to Mrs Board.

Stage 3B: Identify your service needs

Any of the needs assessment exercises in 3A may also reveal service needs.

- Invite the prescribing adviser from the PCO, or a local pharmacist, to review or comment on your management of repeat prescribing arrangements with special emphasis on NSAIDs.
- Pull the notes of everyone receiving repeat prescribing of NSAIDs over the course of six weeks to be sure of catching all relevant patients, to check for any past history of peptic ulcer. If you are a paperless or paperlight practice, you should be able to undertake such a check from your computer records.
- Invite Mrs Board (once she is better) and any other patients who have made justified complaints to work with the practice team to review and critique systems and organisation.

Stage 4: Make and carry out a learning and action plan

*   Read up about the frequency of adverse effects with NSAIDs, contraindications to treatment and best practice in prescribing.[2]
*   Work with the practice team to learn from the significant event audit of Mrs Board's case, and make an action plan to minimise recurrence (e.g. issue a reminder to patients on NSAIDs to consult to review drug therapy if they experience indigestion; ensure that significant past medical history is flagged up on computer or paper-based medical records).
*   Attend a workshop on chronic pain management to learn about the full range of approaches to providing pain relief: their licensed use, relative effectiveness and frequency of adverse effects.

Stage 5: Document your learning, competence, performance and standards of service delivery

*   Make notes of the significant event audit and subsequent action plan.
*   Keep the revised practice prescribing policy and review arrangements for NSAIDs.
*   Keep the report from the pharmaceutical adviser or local pharmacist.
*   Keep a record of the review of patients on NSAIDs and their past medical history (with anonymised patient details for your portfolio).
*   Record the patients' critique of practice systems and organisation and the subsequent action notes.
*   Keep the record of attendance at the workshop on chronic pain management, your reflections on what you have learnt and what you will change once back in the practice.

Box 10.11:   Case study continued

Mrs Board quickly recovered from the gastric ulcer seen at endoscopy, once her *Helicobacter pylori* infection was treated. She did not lodge a complaint and accepted your apology for the oversight of her previous ulcer history. She felt partly responsible for her stomach bleed as she recalled how you had warned her to stop taking the NSAIDs if they triggered indigestion. She had ignored that advice as she thought that suffering indigestion was better than the severe back pain.

Example cycle of evidence 10.3

- Focus: research
- Other relevant focus: clinical care

Box 10.12:   Case study

A new professor of rheumatology has taken up a post at your local university. He has started several research projects. He is actively recruiting patients for his various trials and asks your practice to refer patients to his team. He needs patients with various conditions who suffer from chronic pain as they want to compare the effects of acupuncture with the use of medication. You can see that patients will benefit from the speedy referral process.

This is just an example. Keep your task simple. You could choose three or four cycles of evidence to demonstrate your competence each year.

Stage 1: Select your aspirations for good practice

The excellent GP:

- protects patients' rights and makes sure that they are not disadvantaged by taking part in research
- has information available on laws and requirements (e.g. research ethics) relating to general practice.

Stage 2: Set the standards for your outcomes

Outcomes might include:

- the way learning is applied
- a learnt skill
- a protocol
- a strategy that is implemented
- meeting recommended standards.

- Ensure the practice has a policy for GPs and staff undertaking research.
- Ensure you have library and learning resources for chronic pain management available.

Stage 3A: Identify your learning needs

- Find out if you can easily access paper-based resources (e.g. books or files) or electronic sites describing best practice in management of trigeminal neuralgia, restless legs, or post-herpetic neuralgia in your practice.
- Reflect on whether you are up to date with current requirements for undertaking research or participating in someone else's research study. Decide if you are clear about research governance, what studies require ethics approval, how you obtain your trust's permission to host research, what information patients need before giving their consent to participate in research, etc.

Stage 3B: Identify your service needs

> Any of the needs assessment exercises in 3A may also reveal service needs.

- Compare best practice in treating pain from trigeminal neuralgia, restless legs and post-herpetic neuralgia with the interventions that the university research team are comparing in their research. Seek an independent view (e.g. another specialist from outside the trial) as to whether patients will be disadvantaged by you referring them to the trial, remembering the benefits of a speedy referral process. Alternatively, you could ask to see any peer review already carried out about the proposed research.
- Ask the PCO for a copy of the algorithm describing research governance management systems and guidance on how they affect you. Discuss with others in the practice what systems you need to develop to link into the new NHS requirements.
- Ask several patients to comment on the trial's patient information leaflet to check that it is suitable for patients in your population.

Stage 4: Make and carry out a learning and action plan

- Meet up with the research governance manager for a tutorial on research ethics and research governance systems. Compose a policy for practice staff to fit the legal and NHS requirements.

- Write out what constitutes best practice in treating trigeminal neuralgia, post-herpetic neuralgia and restless legs syndrome. Then compare previous treatment with the next case of each that presents and add notes about any subsequent change of treatment.
- Attend a seminar by the university research team introducing their research plans and put specific questions and queries to the team.
- Compile a list of library or other resources (paper/electronic) your practice needs to buy so that there is sufficient reference material available in relation to chronic pain management and research ethics. Check your choice with the local health librarian if possible and place an order.

Stage 5: Document your learning, competence, performance and standards of service delivery

- Keep a copy of the practice policy on GPs and staff undertaking research.
- List the contents of the reference library in the practice and the resources available in each consulting room (e.g. paper and electronic versions of *Clinical Evidence*[18]).
- Keep a copy of the research ethics approval and details of the research study in which you intend to participate.
- Record the questions and answers from the research seminar.
- Keep the checklist of best practice in treatment of chronic pain in trigeminal neuralgia, post-herpetic neuralgia and restless legs syndrome.

Box 10.13: Case study continued

After your preparations in understanding and preparing for participating in the research study, all goes smoothly. Patients are happy with the information leaflet about the trials and most consent to join in. Nearly all the local GPs and practices co-operate to refer suitable patients so that the research study is sufficiently powerful to be able to provide conclusive evidence of relative benefits of the treatments being compared.

References

1 Bradbury J (2003) Why do men and women feel and react to pain differently? *Lancet.* **361**: 2052–3.

2 Moore A, Edwards J, Barden J *et al.* (eds) *Bandolier's Little Book of Pain.* Oxford University Press, Oxford.

3   Melzack R (1975) The McGill Pain Questionnaire: major properties and scoring methods. *Pain.* **1**: 277–99.

4   Wilkin D, Hallam L and Doggett MA (1992) *Measures of Need and Outcome for Primary Health Care.* Oxford University Press, Oxford.

5   www.painsociety.org/pain_scales.html.

6   Proctor M and Farquhar C (2003) Dysmenorrhoea. *Clinical Evidence.* **9**: 1994–2013. www.clinicalevidence.com.

7   Binder A (2003) Neck pain. *Clinical Evidence.* **9**: 1277–91. www.clinicalevidence.com.

8   van Tulder M and Koes B (2003) Low back pain and sciatica (chronic). *Clinical Evidence.* **9**: 1260–76. www.clinicalevidence.com.

9   Zakrzewska J (2003) Trigeminal neuralgia. *Clinical Evidence.* **9**: 1490–8. www.clinicalevidence.com.

10 Joint Formulary Committee (2003) *British National Formulary.* British Medical Association/Royal Pharmaceutical Society, London.

11 www.rls.org.

12 http://welcome.to/ekbom.

13 Telstad W, Sorensen O, Larsen S *et al.* (1984) Treatment of restless legs syndrome with carbamazepine: a double-blind study. *British Medical Journal.* **288**: 444–6.

14 Macmahon D and Chaudhuri R (2003) Identifying and treating restless legs syndrome. *Prescribing in Practice.* 48–52.

15 Brodeur C, Montplaisir J, Godbout R *et al.* (1988) Treatment of restless legs syndrome and periodic movements during sleep with L-dopa: a double-blind, controlled study. *Neurology.* **38**: 1845–8.

16 Lancaster T, Wareham D and Yaphe J (2003) Postherpetic neuralgia. *Clinical Evidence.* **9**: 890–900.

17 www.neuropathy-trust.org.

18 www.clinicalevidence.com.

And finally

We hope that you have found that the stages in our 'cycle of evidence' are a useful approach to gathering information about what you need to learn. You can also use it to identify improvements you or others need to make to the way you deliver services.

It is easy to feel overwhelmed by the magnitude of the task to demonstrate that you are competent and perform consistently well as a doctor, in order to retain your licence to practise. Remember that you should be producing evidence about the breadth of your practice, every five years. Take your time and select three or four cycles of evidence each year that span several headings of *Good Medical Practice* at one time.[1]

Ask others for help. Your practice manager or the receptionists should be able to help you to collect information about what you need to learn, or about gaps in services. You can delegate much of the administrative side. Your colleagues or your patients will be well placed to help you to set your aspirations for good practice and set achievable standards for your outcomes – of learning and improvements in service delivery. Perhaps your CPD tutor can help you to develop learning and action in your PDP. These cycles of evidence will be the nucleus of your PDP. Colleagues in the team can support you in documenting the evidence of your competence, performance and subsequent standards of service delivery. Other books in this series might help you to look at specific clinical areas, especially those where quality frameworks or special interests require your attention. Remember to visit this book's supporting website, which includes useful website links.[2]

So the evidence will be there ready to submit for appraisal interviews or revalidation, but the results will show what a good doctor you really are. This should give you increasing confidence and self-respect. Enjoy your professional glow.

References

1   General Medical Council (2001) *Good Medical Practice*. General Medical Council, London.

2   http://health.mattersonline.net.

Index